Textbook of
Pharmaceutical
Drug Analysis

Textbook of
Pharmaceutical
Drug Analysis

M. Zaffer Ahmad
Faculty of Pharmacy
Jamia Hamdard (Hamdard University)
Hamdard Nagar, New Delhi

Mohammed Ali
Faculty of Pharmacy
Jamia Hamdard (Hamdard University)
Hamdard Nagar, New Delhi

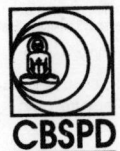

CBSPD

CBS Publishers & Distributors Pvt Ltd

New Delhi • Bengaluru • Chennai • Kochi • Kolkata • Lucknow • Mumbai
Hyderabad • Jharkhand • Nagpur • Patna • Pune • Uttarakhand

A Textbook of
Pharmaceutical Drug Analysis

ISBN: 978-81-239-1675-0

Copyright © Authors and Publisher

First Edition: 2009

Reprint: 2009, 2012, 2016, 2017, 2018, 2019, 2023, 2024, **2025**

Published by **Satish Kumar Jain** and produced by **Varun Jain** for

CBS Publishers & Distributors Pvt Ltd

4819/XI Prahlad Street, 24 Ansari Road, Daryaganj, New Delhi 110 002, India.
Ph: 011-23266838, 23289259   Website: www.cbspd.com
                                e-mail: delhi@cbspd.com
Corporate Office: 204 FIE, Industrial Area, Patparganj, Delhi 110 092
Ph: 011-4934 4934   Fax: 011-4934 4935
                        e-mail: publishing@cbspd.com; publicity@cbspd.com

Branches

- **Bengaluru:** Seema House 2975, 17th Cross, KR Road, Banasankari 2nd Stage, Bengaluru 560 070, Karnataka, India
  Ph: +91-80-26771678/79   Fax: +91-80-26771680   e-mail: bangalore@cbspd.com
- **Chennai:** 18/8B, Subbarayan Street, Shenoy Nagar, Chennai 600 030, Tamil Nadu, India
  Ph: +91-44-42032115, 26681266   e-mail: chennai@cbspd.com
- **Kochi:** 42/1325, 1326, Power House Road, Opp KSEB, Power House, Ernakulum Kochi 682 018, Kerala, India
  Ph: +91-484-4059061-65,67   Fax: +91-484-4059065   e-mail: kochi@cbspd.com
- **Kolkata:** 147, Hind Ceramics Compound, 1st Floor, Nilgunj Road, Belghoria, Kolkata-700056, West Bengal, India
  Ph: +033-25633055, 033-25633056   e-mail: kolkata@cbspd.com
- **Lucknow:** Basement, Khushnuma Complex, 7 Meerabai Marg (Behind Jawahar Bhawan), Lucknow-226001, UP, India
  Ph: +0522-4000032   e-mail: tiwari.lucknow@cbspd.com
- **Mumbai:** PWD Shed, Gala no 25/26, Ramchandra Bhatt Marg, Next to JJ Hospital Gate no. 2, Opp. Union Bank of India, Noorbaug, Mumbai-400009, Maharashtra, India
  Ph: 022-66661880/89   e-mail: mumbai@cbspd.com

Representatives

• Hyderabad	0-9885175004	• Jharkhand	0-9811541605	• Nagpur	0-8692091830
• Patna	0-9334159340	• Pune	0-9664372571	• Uttarakhand	0-9716462459

Printed at Neekunj Print Process, Haryana, India

Preface

Analytical procedures forming the backbone of research and development in science and technology has been the prime objective in preparing this write-up on Text book of Pharmaceutical Drug Analysis. The book is focused on the B.Pharm syllabus, both for theory and practicals, as recommended by the All India Council for Technical Education and adopted by most of the universities in the country.

Pharmaceutical analysis or drug analysis deals with the bulk material, dosage forms, and, more recently, biological samples in support of biopharmaceutical and pharmacokinetic studies, we regard it as a branch of pharmaceutics rather than in pharmaceutical chemistry. The course in pharmaceutical analysis or drug assay retains a place in the undergraduate curriculum, despite its less importance for practising pharmacist. The pharmacist is primarily an expert on drugs, and an important aspect of the development, production, distribution and use of drugs in their analysis.

In this book we try to give sufficiently systematic and detailed account of some important chapters of pharmaceutical analysis to permit the pharmacy students and the pharmacists to understand, principles of analysis and many of them in detail. Our major objective of this text is to provide a thorough background in those analytical principles that are particularly important in pharmaceutical analysis. We aim to teach those laboratory skills that will give students confidence in their ability to obtain experimental data.

The subject matter is discussed in 8 chapters covering mainly titrimetry and gravimetry besides general introduction to pharmaceutical analysis. The material in this text covers both fundamental and practical aspects of pharmaceutical analysis. An appendix containing the indicators and equivalant weights of some compounds have also been included. Glossary of important definitions at the end of the book will serve the purpose of quick memory and reference. The section demanding more interpretation and attention can be taken care of in the next revised edition. Hence the comments and suggestions from the readers regarding the relevent improvements in the book are always welcome.

Though the best of efforts have been attempted to avoid errors yet possibility of any printing error or otherwise due to oversight cannot be overruled. Readers ar requested to point out the same for the purpose of rectification.

We didn't claim any originality of matter and wish to express our indebtness to the authors of various reference books and literature for collecting important information included in the present manuscript whose work has been individually cited and duly acknowledged. Our sincere vote of thanks goes to Dr. U. K. Bajaj and Mr. Muneeb-U-Rehman for sparing the valuable time to provide the immense support to this effort. Our greatest depth of gratitude is due to Sh. Satish Kumar Jain and Vinod Kumar Jain, CBS Publishers and Distributors, for continuous courtesy and full co-operation in bringing out the book of our satisfaction and Mr. Anurag Trivedi for setting the pages in perfect format.

Finally, we express our deep gratitude to our family members and friends for being supportive in times of stress in bringing out this book. No major professional project can be completed without co-opration and encouragement of one's family.

M.Zaffer Ahmad
Mohammed Ali

Contents

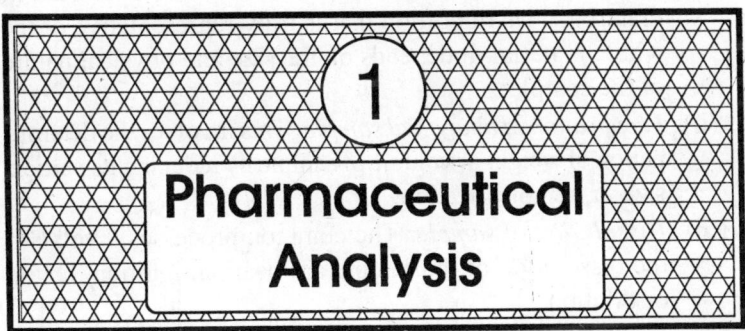

Pharmaceutical Analysis

Pharmaceutical analysis refers to the chemical analysis of drug molecules or medicinal agents and their metabolites. It consists of the estimation of the quality and quantity of drugs and fine chemicals, which are used in pharmaceutical preparations.

Pharmaceutical Analysis Generally Involves Two Steps

- Separation of the compound of interest.
- Quantification of the compound.

Scope

The scope of the pharmaceutical analysis can be extended by incorporating the analysis of the chemical constituents during disease states which serves as a diagnostic aid in the practice of medicine.

1.1 Methods of Pharmaceutical or Drug Analysis

(1) Chemical Method of Analysis

The study deals with the application of process or series of processes in order to identify a substance or complex compound, the components of a solution or a mixture, or the determination of the structures of chemical compounds.

Stages in a Chemical Analysis

   (i) *Sampling:* The process of withdrawing from the bulk of material, a small portion that is truly representative of the whole material. It depends on the size and physical nature of the sample.

  (ii) *Preparation of analytical sample:* This involves the determination of weight or volume of sample by reducing its particle size or homogenization.

 (iii) *Dissolution of sample:* The common processes involve in the dissolution of the sample are heating, ignition, fusion or dilution.

 (iv) *Removal of impurities:* This can be done either by filtration, crystallization or chromatographic techniques.

  (v) *Measurement of sample:* This procedure of the sample includes calibration, standardization and validation.

 (vi) *Results:* This involves the calculation of analytical results, stastically evaluation of data and the presentation of data.

Types of Chemical Analysis

Depending upon the site of approach of a given substance, chemical analysis may be of two types;

(i) Qualitative analysis

Chemical analysis dealing with the study of nature or quality of the compound or mixture is called qualitative analysis. It involves the identification of constituent radicals present in the inorganic mixture and presence or absence of particular element, and functional group in an organic compound.

(ii) Quantitative analysis

Chemical analysis dealing with the study of determination of how much of each component or of specified compound is present in a given sample. The testing of a substance or mixture to determine the amounts and proportions of its chemical constituents is called quantitative analysis.

When a completely unknown sample is presented to an analyst, the first requirement is usually to determine which substances are present in it. This fundamental problem may be faced in deciding the nature of impurities present in a given sample. After determining the nature of the constituents of given sample, the analyst then finds out the amount of each component, or of specified components. Such determinations are a part of quantitative analysis, and a variety of techniques are available to supply the required information.

Significances of the quantitative analysis: The significances of the quantitative analysis are enlisted as:

(a) It will be necessary to ascertain the composition of the mixture which shows the optimum characteristics for the purpose for which the product or drug has been developed.

(b) Since the value of the raw material may be governed by the amount of the required ingredient it contains, a quantitative analysis is performed to establish the proportion of the essential component. Raw material is examined to ensure that there are no unusual substances present that might upset the manufacturing process or appear as a harmful impurity in the final product. Furthermore; this procedure is often called as **assaying.**

(c) The final manufacture product is subjected to quality control to ensure that its essential components are present within a permitted range of composition, whereas impurities do not exceed certain specified limits.

(d) In hospitals, chemical analysis is widely used to assist in the diagnosis of illness and in monitoring the condition of patients. Chemical tests for determination of sugars, bile acids, proteins, uric acid and sterols are helpful in diagnosis.

(e) In farming, the nature and level of fertilizer application is based on information obtained by analyzing the soil to determine its content of the essential plant nutrients nitrogen, phosphorus and potassium, and the trace elements required for healthy plant growth.

Types of Quantitative Analysis

(i) Titrimetry

A quantitative method of analysis dealing with the volumes of solution and their measurements is termed as titrimetric analysis or titrimetry. The substance is allowed to react with an appropriate reagent added as a standard solution and the volume of the solution needed for complete reaction is determined. The common types of reactions that are used in titrimetry are:

(a) *Neutralization (acid-base) reactions:* Acid-base titration is based on the neutralization reaction between the analyte and an acidic or basic titrant. These reactions use a pH indicator, a pH meter, or a conductance meter to determine the end point.

(b) *Precipitation reactions:* A precipitation titration comprises a class of reactions that requires a formation of insoluble precipitate, provided that the end point at which the precipitation is complete, can be determined.

(c) *Oxidation-reduction reactions:* A redox titration is based on an oxidation-reduction reaction between the analyte and an oxidant or reductant. A potentiometer or a redox indicator is used to determine the end point. Frequently either the reactants or the titrant have a color intense enough that an additional indicator is not needed.

(d) *Complex forming reactions:* A complexometric titration is based on the formation of a complex between the analyte and the titrant. The chelating agent EDTA is very commonly used to titrate metal ions in solution. These titrations generally require specialized indicators that form weaker complexes with the analyte. A common example is Eriochrome T for the titration of calcium and magnesium ions.

(e) *Non-aqueous titration:* Non-aqueous titration is the titration of substances dissolved in nonaqueous solvents. It is the most common titrimetric procedure used in pharmacopoeial assays and serves a double purpose:

   • It is suitable for the titration of very weak acids and bases, and
   • It provides a solvent in which organic compounds are soluble.

(ii) Gravimetry

It involves the separation of the constituents to be estimated in the form of an insoluble precipitate. The insoluble precipitate is washed to free it from all impurities, dried and weighed either as such or ignited to leave a residue of some other compound which is then weighed. Now from its weight and known composition, the amount of the constituent in the given sample is calculated, e.g.; determination of chlorine content in common salt (NaCl). The various forms of gravimetry are;

   (a) *Electrogravimetry:* involves electrolysis and the material deposited on one of the electrodes is weighed.

   (b) *Thermogravimetry (TG):* estimates the change in weight as a function of temperature.

   (c) *Differential thermal analysis:* (DTA) determines the difference in temperature between a test substance and an inert reference material.

   (d) *Differential scanning colorimetry (DSC):* Records the energy needed to establish a zero temperature differende between a test substance and a reference material.

(iii) Volumetry

It is concerned with measuring the volume of gas evolved and absorbed in a chemical method.

(2) Physical Method of Analysis

It involves the determination of physical properties of liquids like specific gravity, viscosity or surface tension. The common types of measurements that are used in physical method of analysis are:

   (i) *Refractometry:* It involves the measurement of refractive index of liquids using a refractometer. For example, refractive index of arachis oil against water.

   (ii) *Polarimetry:* It is used to measure optical rotation of an optically active compound using a polarimeter. For example, optical rotation of sucrose.

   (iii) *Viscometery:* It involves the measurement of viscosity of a liquid using viscometer. For example viscosities of solvents like ethanol and carbon tetrachloride.

(3) Electrical Methods of Analysis

It involves the measurement of current, voltage or resistance in relation to the concentration of a certain species in solution. The common types of measurements that are used in electrical methods of analysis include:

   (i) *Voltametry:* It involves the measurement of current at a micro electrode at specified voltage.

  (ii) *Coulometry:* It measures current and time needed to complete an electrochemical reaction or to generate sufficient material to react completely with a specified reagent.

 (iii) *Potentiometry:* It is used to measure the potential of an electrode in equilibrium with an ion to be determined.

(4) Spectroscopic Methods of Analysis

Spectral methods measure the electromagnetic radiation that is absorbed, scattered, or emitted by the analyte. The methods of measurement of radiation vary from one method to another. The important spectral methods are:

   (i) *Absorption spectroscopy:* It depends on measuring the amount of radiant energy of a particular wave length absorbed by the sample. Absorption methods are usually classified according to wavelengths involved as visible, ultraviolet or infrared spectroscopy. The visible spectrophotometry is sometimes called as ***colorimetry***.

  (ii) *Turbidimetric and nephelometric methods:* These procedures are used to measure the amount of light stopped or scattered by a suspension.

 (iii) *Emission spectroscopy:* It determines the amount of radiant energy of a particular wavelength emitted by the sample.

 (iv) *Flame photometry:* It uses a solution of the sample injected into a flame.

  (v) *Fluorimetry:* It takes a suitable substance in solution (commonly a metal-fluorescent reagent complex) and excites it using visible or ultra violet radiation.

(5) Chromatographic Methods

These methods are used to separate mixtures of substances and to identify components of a mixture. For example paper chromatography, thin layer chromatography and gas-liquid chromatography.

(6) Special Techniques

(i) *X-ray methods:* X-rays are produced when high-speed electrons collide with a solid target (which can be the material under investigation). It is possible to identify certain emission peaks that are characteristic of elements contained in the target.

(ii) *Radioactivity:* This procedure measures intensity of the radiation from a naturally occurring radioactive material; measuring radioactivity induced by exposing the sample to a neutron source (activation analysis) or isotope dilution and radio immunoassay.

(iii) *Kinetic methods:* These methods are based on increasing the speed of a reaction by adding a small amount of a catalyst, within limits, and the rate of the catalyzed reaction will be governed by the amount of catalyst present.

1.2 Volumetric Analysis

Volumetric analysis depends on the measurement of the volumes of solution of the interacting substances. In this analysis a measured volume of solution of a substance is allowed to react completely with the solution of given strength of another substance. The end point of the reaction is indicated by some marked changes such as appearance or disappearance of color or formation of precipitate and the process is termed as *titration*. The stage during titration at which the reaction is just complete is known as the *equivalence* or *end point*. Generally end point in a volumetric analysis is detected by the addition of a suitable substance called *indicator* that changes its color when the reaction is just completed.

Fundamentals of Volumetric Analysis

The fundamental requirements to carry out titrimetric or volumetric processes are:

(i) The reactions between titrate and titrant must be well defined, i.e., definite amounts of reactants must react to produce definite amounts of products.

(ii) The reaction must be rapid so that little time is needed to complete the titration. A catalyst may also be used to increase the rate of the reaction.

(iii) Titrimetric calculations are based on 100% reaction between the reactants, thus mixing of equivalents amounts of the reactions must give a complete reactions.

(iv) A standard solution of reagent, i.e., *titrant* should be taken in a burette and *titrate* is kept in a conical flask as shown in Fig.1.1.

(v) An *indicator* kept in conical flask must be available to show the completion of the reaction.

(vi) The end point should be well defined.

(vii) The volume of titrant used for completion of reaction is known as *titre value*.

(viii) As the concentration of the reagent solution is known, the quantity of reagent present in the solution can be calculated.

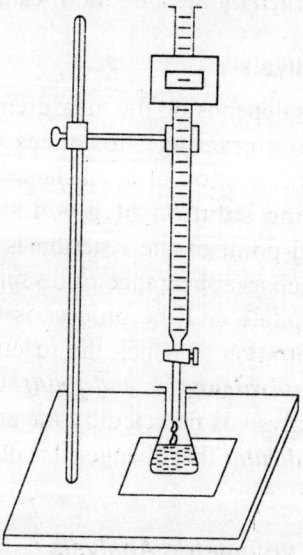

Fig.1.1: Titration setup: *The titrant drops from the burette into the analyte solution in the flask. An indicator present then changes color permanently at the endpoint.*

Steps Involved in Volumetric Analysis

The volumetric determination of a solution of a given substance (analyte) with the reagents involves the following steps:

(i) A known amount of substance is dissolved in a known volume of water so that the concentration of the reagent solution can be calculated. Such a solution is known as *standard solution* and this solution is prepared in a volumetric flask.

(ii) A known volume of the analyte solution is taken in a conical flask with the help of a pipette. The analyte solution is also called as sample solution, test solution or titrate solution.

(iii) Few drops of an indicator are added to the titrant solution taken in the conical flask. The use of the indicator is to show the color change when the reaction between the analyte and the reagent solution is just complete.

(iv) The objective of titrating an alkaline solution with a standard solution of an acid is to determine the amount of acid which is exactly equivalent chemically to the amount of the base present. This point of neutralization is termed as *equivalence point* or theoretical end point due to formation of salt.

Volumetric Apparatus

Apparatus used for titrations are called *volumetric apparatus* due to involvement of measurements of volumes. Acid-base titrations form part of a group of laboratory procedures known as volumetric analysis. Some of the apparatus are given as:

1. Pipette: A bulb pipette is designed to deliver an accurately known volume of solution, after it has been filled exactly to the mark. They are available in volumes of 1, 2, 5, 10, and 20 ml. All volumetric pipettes are calibrated in units of milliliters (ml). The pipette is held vertically to fix the mark at the same level as the eye. The withdrawing of solution by pipette and reading of pipette are shown in Fig. 1.2.

Pipettes are of Two Types

(i) *Transfer pipettes:* Which have one mark and withdraw a small and constant volume of the solution; and

(ii) *Measuring or graduated pipettes:* Which are graduated and used to deliver various small volumes.

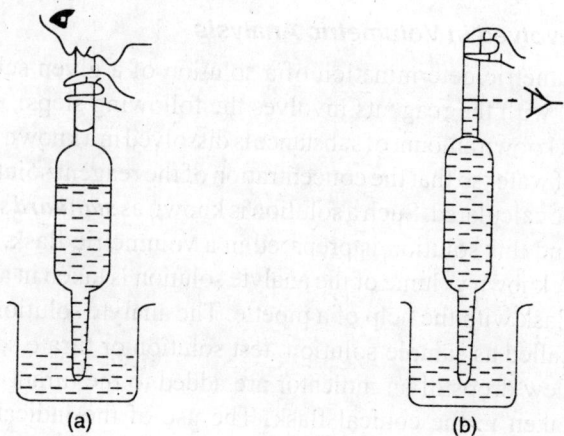

Fig. 1.2: *Withdrawing of solution by the pipette (a) and reading of pipette (b)*

During withdrawel the adhering drops at the tip are removed by stroking against an inside walls of glass surface or touching to the surface of solution.

2. Beaker: It is a container having beak like structure. A borosil beaker is used as it can withstand with frequent heating and cooling. Beakers of different capacities, e.g., 50 ml, 100 ml, 500 ml and 1000 ml are available in market. The following processes are carried out in such container:

  (i) Preparation of solution.

  (ii) Heating.

  (iii) Precipitation.

3. Burette: A burette consists of a graduated tube fitted with a stopcock and is used to deliver variable volumes. Burettes are normally available in maximum capacities of 2, 5, 10, 25, 50 and 100 ml. Before using, the burette is thoroughly cleaned with a cleaning agent, rinsed well with distilled water; the stopcock is lubricated and fixed in a burette holder. The solution is filled with the help of a small funnel up to zero mark. The liquid is discharged from a burette into a conical flask. The flask is gently rotated with the right hand for mixing the contents well. *Meniscus* is a curve in the surface of a liquid and is produced in response to the surface of the container or another object. It can be either concave or convex

Fig. 1.3. A convex meniscus occurs when the molecules of the liquid repel the molecules of the container or object. This may be seen between mercury and glass in barometers. Conversely, a concave meniscus occurs when the molecules of the liquid attract those of the container. This can be seen between water and glass.

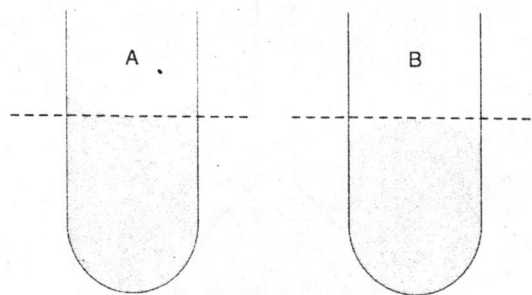

Fig. 1.3: Meniscus
A: This bottom of a concave meniscus.
B: The top of a convex meniscus.

Reading a Burette

Assume that the burette is filled to the point indicated in the Fig. 1.4 at the right. You would record the initial point as 26.40 ml; the ending point would be 26.80 ml. Remember that you should read the number that is at the bottom of the meniscus.

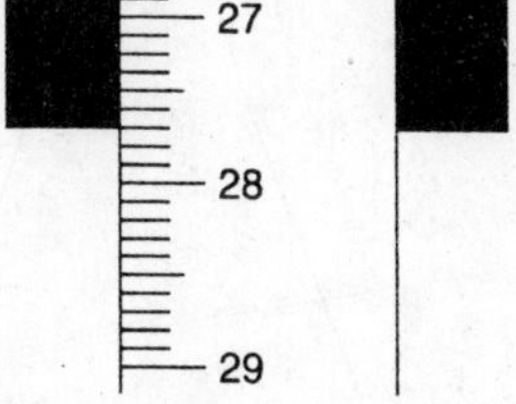

Fig. 1.4: Reading of burette

4. Conical flask: A conical flask is a flat-bottomed pear-shaped apparatus with short narrow neck. A thin line mark around the neck indicates the volume that it holds at a certain definite temperature. Solutions to be titrated are usually pipetted into a conical flask, also known as an Erlenmeyer flask (Fig. 1.6).

5. Volumetric flask: These flasks are used to prepare standard solutions of solutes. A known mass of solute is placed in a flask, dissolved in pure water, and then made up to a mark etched in the neck of the flask. Volumetric flasks are normally supplied in volumes of 100 ml to 1000 ml. [Fig. 1.5]

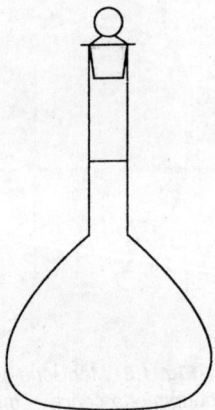

Fig.1.5: Volumetric flask

6. Measuring cylinder: These are used to measure standard solutions of solutes. With permanent graduations they are made

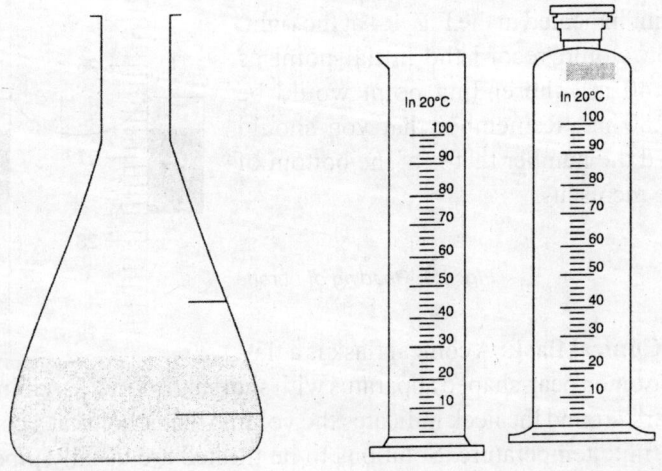

Fig.1.6: An Erlenmeyer flask   *Fig. 1.7:* Measuring cylinder

up of borosilicate glass. The commonly used sizes of measuring cylinder are 10 ml, 50 ml, 100 ml, 250 ml, 500 ml, and 1000 ml. Before use, the burette is thoroughly cleaned with a cleaning agent, rinsed well with distilled water. While reading the measuring cylinder, remember that you should read the number that is at the bottom of the meniscus. [Fig. 1.7]

Some Important Terms in Volumetric Analysis

1. Titrand or titrate: It is prepared by dissolving a known amount of substance into known amount of water or solvent. It is prepared in volumetric flask, it has exact purity, non hygroscopic in nature. It is also known primary standard solution, test solution or analyte solution.

2. Titrant: The secondary standard solution is known as titrant. It is used in the process of standardization and whose content or concentration of active compound is found by comparison against primary standard. It is prepared in graduated volumetric flask and taken in burette.

3. Indicator: Indicator is an organic dye which signals the completion of reaction or titration by the visual change in the color, e.g., methyl orange, phenolphthalein, starch and phenol red.

4. Equivalence point: It is the point of a reaction or titration when the number of titrant molecules reacting with titrate molecules will be equal.

5. Standardization: It is the process whereby the concentration of one solution is determined by the known concentration of the other solution.

6. End point: It is the exact stage at which an indicator gives its visual color change and the reaction is just complete.

1.3 Standard Solution

A solution whose concentration is accurately known is called a standard solution.

Preparation: An exactly weighed amount of the substance, of definite and known composition is dissolved in distilled water and made up to known volume in a graduated volumetric flask. From the known weight and volume, the concentration of the solution is calculated. Various substances used for making standard solution in volumetric analysis are classified in the following types as:

1. Primary Standard: A primary standard is a compound of sufficient purity from which a standard solution can be prepared by direct weighing of a quantity of it and followed by detection to give a defined volume of solution, the solution then produced is a primary standard solution.

A primary standard should satisfy the following requirements:

  (i) It must be easy to purify, to dry (preferably at $110°–120°C$) and to preserve in a pure state.

 (ii) The substance should not to be altered in air during weighing, this condition implies that it should not be hygroscopic, oxidized by air, or affected by CO_2 the standard should mention an unchanged composition during storage.

(iii) The substance should be capable of being tested for impurities by qualities and other tests of known sensitivity. (The total amount of impurity should not exceed 0.01–0.02%).

 (iv) The substance should be readily soluble under each condition in which it is employed.

  (v) The reaction with the standard solution should be stiochoimetric: quantitative relationship between reactants and products in a chemical reaction.

Some examples of primary standards are:

  (a) Arsenic trioxide for standardization of iodine and cerium (iv) sulfate solutions.

  (b) Benzoic acid for standardization of TBAH (Tetra butyl ammonium hydrate) in methanol solutions.

  (c) Potassium bromate ($KBrO_3$) for standardization of sodium thiosulphate solutions.

  (d) Potassium hydrogen phthalate (usually called KHP) and unhydrated oxalic acid for standardization of sodium hydroxide and perchloric acid in acetic acid solutions.

  (e) Sodium carbonate for standardization of hydrochloric, sulfuric and nitric acid solutions.

(f) Sodium chloride for standardization of silver nitrate solutions.

(g) Sulfanilic acid for standardization of sodium nitrite solutions.

(h) Zinc powder for standardization of EDTA solutions.

2. Secondary standard: A secondary standard is a substance which may be used for standardization, and whose content of the active substance has been found by comparison against a primary standard. They are prepared in a laboratory for specific analysis and are usually standardized against primary standard. It follows that a secondary standard solution is a solution in which the concentration of dissolved solute has not been determined from the weight of the compound dissolved but by reaction (titration) of measured volume of a primary standard solution.

The commonly used secondary standards are:

Alkali hydroxides → Potassium hydroxide (KOH) and sodium hydroxide (NaOH)

Mineral acids → Hydrochloric acid (HCl), sulphuric acid (H_2SO_4) and nitric acid (HNO_3)

Oxidizing agent → Potassium permanganate ($KMnO_4$) and potassium dichromate ($K_2Cr_2O_7$)

The secondary standard component which is not obtained in pure state, e.g., caustic soda (NaOH) and mineral acids (HCl, H_2SO_4 and HNO_3) are prepared little more concentrated than the required and to dilute it with distilled water until the desired normality is obtained. The solution must be standardized and for standardization they has to be titrated against the solution of pure substances of known concentration (primary standard).

1.4 Methods of Expressing Concentration

Concentration is the measure of how much of a given substance there is mixed with another substance. To concentrate a solution, one must add more solute, or reduce the amount of solvent (for instance, by selective evaporation). By contrast, to dilute a solution, one must add more solvent, or reduce the amount of solute.

The concentration of standard solution in volumetric analysis is often expressed in terms of *titre*, which is the number of grams of substance contained in 1 ml of solution. The titre of H_2SO_4 solution is 0.0049 g/ml which means that each ml of H_2SO_4 solution contains 0.0049 g of H_2SO_4. It is denoted by letter T and for H_2SO_4 is given as:

$$T_{H_2SO_4} = 0.0049 \text{ g/ml}$$

There are various methods of expressing concentration or strength of the solution. The most common are listed below:

(1) Normality: The normality (symbol N) is defined as the number of gram equivalents of the solute per liter of solution.

$$\text{Normality (N)} = \frac{\text{No. of gram equivalents of solute } (n)}{\text{Volume of solution in liters } (v)}$$

The **gram equivalent** of a substance is the number of grams of the substance chemically equivalent to 1 gram-atom (or gram-ion) of hydrogen in a given reaction. To find out the gram equivalents we must write down the reaction equation and calculate how many grams of the substance correspond to 1 gram-atom (or gram-ion) of hydrogen in the reaction. For example, in the equation.

$$HCl + KOH = KCl + H_2O$$
$$CH_3COOH + NaOH = CH_3COONa + H_2O$$

The gram equivalent is one gram-molecule (36.46 g) of HCl and one gram-molecule (60.05 g) of CH_3COOH, because these are the weights of the respective acids which yield one gram-ion of hydrogen, reacting with the hydroxyl ions of the alkali in the reactions. The milligram equivalent is also often used in analytical chemistry. The milligram equivalent (mg-eq) is one-thousands of the gram equivalent, and represents the equivalent weight of a substance expressed in milligrams. For example, 1 g-eq of HCl is 36.46 g.To make clear distinction between grams and gram equivalents, when making a solution with a given molarity, you measure grams of a compound and dissolve them in a known volume. When making a solution with a given normality, you measure gram equivalents of a compound, in grams, and dissolve them in a known volume.

One **normal solution** is a solution which contain one gram equivalent of solute per liter of the solution. Solutions of strengths other than one normal are designated appropriately, e.g.

Twice normal	2 N
Half normal	0.5 N or N/2
Deci-normal	0.1 N or N/10
Centi-normal	0.01 N or N/100

Preparation of 1 N Solution of NaOH (Sodium Hydroxide)

Molecular weight of the NaOH = 40

$$\text{Equivalent weight of the NaOH} = \frac{\text{Molecular weight}}{\text{No. of OH group present}}$$

$$= 40/1$$
$$= 40 \text{ g}$$

Thus, if 40 g of NaOH (Eq. wt. = 40) be dissolved in one liter of solution, normality of the solution is 1 N (one-normal). A solution containing 4.0 g of NaOH is 1/10 N or 0.1 N or *deci normal*.

Preparation of 1 N Solution of Anhydrous Oxalic Acid

Molecular weight of oxalic acid (HOOC-COOH) = 90

Eq. wt = 90/2 = 45

Thus, if 45 g of oxalic acid (Eq. wt. = 45) be dissolved in one liter of distilled water, normality of the solution is one and the solution is called **1 N (one-normal)**.

(2) Molarity: Molarity (symbol M) is defined as the number of moles of solute per liter of solution. If n is the number of moles of solute and v liters the volume of solution.

$$\text{Molarity (M)} = \frac{\text{No. of moles of solute } (n)}{\text{Volume in liters } (v)}$$

For one mole of solute dissolved in one litre of solution M = 1, i.e., molarity is one. Such a solution is called **1 M** ("one molar"). As evident from above expression, unit of molarity is mol/litre or mol/litre^{-1}.

(3) Molality (*m*): The number of moles of the solute per 1000 g of the solvent is called molality of the solution. The SI unit for molality is mol/kg.

$$\text{Molarity } (m) = \frac{\text{No. of moles of solute } (n)}{\text{Volume in kg } (v)}$$

(4) Formality (F): The number of gram formula weight of solute dissolved in one litre of solution is known as formality of that solution.

It is calculated based on the formula weights of chemicals per liter of solution. The difference between formal and molar concentrations is that the formal concentration indicates moles of the original chemical formula in solution, without regard for the species that actually exist in solution.

Molar concentration, on the other hand, is the concentration of species in solution. For example: if one dissolves sodium carbonate (Na_2CO_3) in one litre of water, the compound dissociates into the Na^+ and CO_3^{2-} ions. Some of the CO_3^{2-} reacts with the water to form HCO_3^- and H_2CO_3. If the pH of the solution is low, there is practically no Na_2CO_3 left in the solution. So, although we have added 1 mol of Na_2CO_3 to the solution, it does not contain 1 M of that substance. Rather, it contains a molarity based on the other constituents of the solution. However, one can still say that the solution contains 1 F of Na_2CO_3.

Equivalent Weight (Eq. wt)

The equivalent weight of a substance is defined as the parts by weight of that substance which is chemically equivalent to 1.008 parts by weight of hydrogen or 8 parts by weight of oxygen or 35.45 parts by weight of chlorine. Equivalent weight of the substance is not a constant quantity but its value depends upon the reaction in which it is taking part. The equivalent weight of different substances is determined as:

1. **Eq.wt of an element** $= \dfrac{\text{Atomic weight}}{\text{Valency}}$

2. **Eq.wt of an acid** $= \dfrac{\text{Molecular weight}}{\text{Basicity of acid}}$

Basicity of an acid is considered to be the number of the replaceable hydrogen atoms present in it.

or equivalent weight of acid $= \dfrac{\text{Molar mass of the acid}}{\text{No. of replaceable hydrogen atoms}}$

For example in HCl, the number of replaceable hydrogen is 1.
Molar mass of the acid = 36.5
Equivalent weight of acid = 36.5/1 = 36.5

3. Eq.wt of Base $= \dfrac{\text{Molecular weight}}{\text{Acidity of base}}$

Acidity of a base is considered to be number of replaceable hydroxyl ions present in it.

Equivalent weight of bases like sodium carbonate (Na_2CO_3) or potassium carbonate (K_2CO_3)

$$\text{Eq. wt} = \dfrac{\text{Molar mass of the salt}}{\text{Total charge on metallic ions on that base}}$$

Na_2CO_3	$=$	Na^{+2}	$=$ Charge $= (2)$	$106/2 = 53$
K_2CO_3	$=$	K^{+2}	$=$ Charge $= (2)$	$138/2 = 69$
$NaHCO_3$	$=$	Na^{+2}	$=$ Charge $= (1)$	$84/1 = 84$
$KHCO_3$	$=$	K^{+}	$=$ Charge $= (1)$	$100/1 = 100$

Table 1.1: Equivalent weights of some compounds

Name of compound and their formulae	Molecular weight	Acidity/Basic/ loss or gain of electron	Equivalent weight
Hydrochloric acid (HCl)	36.46	1	36.46
Nitric acid (HNO_3)	63.01	1	63.01
Sulphuric acid (H_2SO_4)	98.07	2	49.03
Acetic acid (CH_3COOH)	60.05	1	60.05
Boric acid (H_3BO_3)	61.83	3	20.16
Sodium hydroxide (NaOH)	40.0	1	40.00
Potassium hydroxide (KOH)	56.11	1	56.11
Sodium carbonate (Na_2CO_3)	105.99	2	53.00

Table 1.1 (Contd.)

Sodium bicar-bonate ($NaHCO_3$)	84.01	1	84.01
Potassium car-bonate (K_2CO_3)	138.21	2	69.10
Potassium permanganate ($KMmO_4$)	158.03	5	31.60
Potassium dichromate ($K_2Cr_2O_7$)	294.18	6	49.03
Iodine (I_2)	253.8	2	126.90
Oxalic acid anhydrous ($COOH)_2$	90.0	2	45.00
Oxalic acid dihydrate $(COOH)_2.2H_2O$	126.07	2	63.03
Sodium thiosulphate $Na_2S_2O_3.5H_2O$	248.17	1	248.17

Relation of Different Concentration Terms Used in Volumetric Analysis

1. Strength (g / l) = Normality × equivalent weight.
2. Normality = Molarity × change in oxidation number.
3. No. of equivalents = Normality × volume (l)
4. No. of equivalents = $\dfrac{\text{Weight in grams}}{\text{Equivalent weight}}$
5. Equivalent weight of acid

   $= \dfrac{\text{Molar mass of the acid}}{\text{No. of replaceable hydrogen atoms}}$
6. Equivalent weight of base

   $= \dfrac{\text{Molar mass of the base}}{\text{No. of replaceable hydroxyl atoms}}$

1.5 Accuracy

The accuracy of a determination may be defined as the closeness of a measured valve to the true or most probable value. For analytical methods there are two possible ways of determining the accuracy, viz; absolute method and comparative method.

1. **Absolute method:** The test of accuracy of the method under consideration is carried out by taking varying amounts of the constituents and proceeding according to specified instructions. The amount of the constituent must be varied, because the determinate errors in the procedure may be a function of the amount used. The difference between the mean of an adequate number of results and the amount of the constituent actually present is a measure of the accuracy of the method in the absence of the foreign substance. Here primary standards are used.

2. **Comparative method:** In this method of accuracy the solid synthetic secondary standard samples of desired composition are prepared. The samples are resorted further so as to determine the content of the constituents by one or more accurate method of analysis. This method indicates the absence of appreciable systematic error in the procedure of analysis.

1.6 Precision

Precision is defined at the concordance or agreement of a series of measurement of the same quantity. When an analyst is able to reproduce two or more measurement with only slight difference in the results, his work may be reproduced as to be précised. In short the precision is the reproducibility of a measurement.

There are two forms of precision;

1. **Run precision repeatability:** If an analyst has made the determination on the same day in rapid successions, the set of results would be defined as repeatable.

2. **Run precision reproducibility:** If an analyst has made the determination on the separate days when laboratory condition may vary, the set of results would be defined as reproducible.

Precision measures

(i) *Mean or average:* Mean or average is obtained by dividing the sum of a set of measurements by the number of individual results in the set.

$$\text{Mean, } m = \frac{M_n}{n}$$

Where M is the individual measurement and n is the total no. of measurement.

(ii) *Mean deviation of a single measurement:* It is the mean of the deviations of all the individual measurements. It can be calculated as:

(a) Determining the arithmetic mean of results,

(b) Calculating the deviation of each individual's measurement from the mean,

(c) Dividing the sum of deviation (regardless of sign), by the number of measurements and

(d) Coefficient of variable (CV) $= \dfrac{S \times 100}{x}$

S = Standard deviation

x = Mean

$$\text{Mean deviation} = \overline{d} \; \frac{|M_n - n|}{x}$$

Where, $\overline{d} \rightarrow$ Absolute value of deviation of the M_n^{th} number from the mean.

(iii) *Relative mean deviation (RMD):* It is the mean deviation divided by the mean and expressed in % percentage or parts per mellion (ppm).

$$\text{RMD} = \frac{\text{Mean deviation}}{\text{Mean}} \times 100$$

(iv) *Standard deviation (S)*

$$\partial = \frac{(M_n - m)^2}{n}$$

When no. of determination is smaller the above equation is modified as:

$$\delta = \frac{(M_n - m)^2}{(n - 1)}$$

(v) *Variance (V):* It is square of standard deviation (*S*).
$$V = S^2$$

Illustration of Precision and Accuracy

To explain the phenomenon of precision and accuracy let us take a substance contain $49.10 \pm 0.02\%$ of a constituent *x*. On the same sample, work was done by two analyst and following results were obtained. The results were,

Analyst I	Analyst II
percentage of *x*	percentage of *x*
49.01%	49.40%
49.25%	49.44%
49.08 %	49.42 %
49.14 %	49.43 %

The results of analyst I range from 49.01% to 49.25% and the mean is given as;

$$\frac{a + b}{2} = 49.12\%$$

This is very close to the actual amount *x* present in an original substance.

The results of analyst II range from 49.40 % to 49.44% and the mean is given as;

$$\frac{a + b}{2} = 49.42\%$$

This is very much different from actual amount *x* present in an original substance. The precision is inferior to the results given by the analyst II. Therefore, values obtained by the analyst II are very precise but not very accurate. It is apparent that there is a constant (systematic) error present in the result of analyst II. Therefore, values obtained by the analyst I are not precise but very accurate.

Table 1.2: *Difference between precision and accuracy.*

Precision	Accuracy
The concordant of a series of measurement of same quantity.	The degree of agreement different between the observed or measured value of true or most probable value.
Express reproducibility of a measurement.	Express correctness of a measurement.
High degree of precision does not imply accuracy.	Accuracy without precession is impossible.
The pression of an assay in inherent in the analytical method, but may be modified by the sensitivity of any instrument used and skill of the analyst.	Accuracy can be established by concurrence of results obtained in two or make indepedent analytical methods where the accuracy of one method isestablished, the accuracy of the other method can also be established.

1.7 Significant Figures

A figure or digit denotes any one of the ten numerals (e.g., 0, 1, 2, 3, 4, 5, 6, 7, 8 and 9). A figure or digit alone or in combination serves to express a *number*. A significant figure is a digit having some practical meaning, i.e., it is a figure or digit which denotes the amount of quantity in the place in which it stands or the digit of a number which are needed to express the precision of the measurements from which the number derived are known as significant figures.

(i) 1.3680 and 1.008]2 g → Five significant figures.
(ii) 0.0035 and 0.0025 g   → Two significant figures.
(iii) 0.456, and 456 g   → Three significant figures.

Significant figure are all the figures in a number apart from zero, on the left, or of zeros on the right if these replace unknown figures or are written when the number is rounded off. In the quantifies 1.2680 g and 1.0062 g the zero is significant, but in the quantity

0.0025 kg the zeros are not significant figures; they serve only to locate the decimal point and can be omitted by proper choice of units, i.e., 2.5 g. The first two numbers contain 5 significant figures, but 0.0025 contains only 2 significant figures.

(i) 1.2680 g

In quantity 1.2680, the number of significant figures is 5 because zero is significant here and indicates an accuracy of 0.1 mg.

(ii) 1.0062 g

1.0062 g contains 5 significant figures because two zeros within a number are significant as they express the exact quantity.

(iii) 0.0025 g

0.0025 g contains only 2 significant figures because here the zeros are net significant figures since the zeros in 0.0025 serve only to locate decimal point and can be emitted by the use of proper units like 2.5 mg.

The zeros in the number 7.2500 are significant if they are obtained by weighing on an analytical balance to a precision of 0.0001-0.0002 g. Significant figures must be distinguished from decimal places, e.g., the number 0.0035 has 4 decimal places and 2 significant figures.

Computation Rules for Calculating Significant Figures

Rule 1: In expressing an experimental measurement, never retain more than one doubtful digit. Eliminate all the digits that are not significant.

Rule 2: Retain only significant figures in a result or in any data otherwise it will give only uncertain figures, e.g.; a volume between 30. 5 ml and 30.7 ml should be written as 30.6 ml and not as 30.60 ml as it would be between 30.59 ml and 30.61 ml.

Rule 3: Two rules are given for rejecting superfluous digits;

(i) When the last digit dropped is greater than 5, the last digit retained is increased by one. It is called **rounding up**.

8.492 g → New value will be 8.49 as 2 is smaller than 5.

4.863 g → New value will be 4.9 as 8 is greater than 5.

(ii) When the last digit discarded is less than 5, the last digit retained is decreased by one. It is called **rounding down**.

When the number 5.64987 is rounded to two digits, we get 5.6 as first digit, discarded is 4, which is less than 5.

Rule 4: In addition there should be in each number only as many significant figures as there are in the least accurately known number. The result should be reported with the same number of decimal places as that of the term with the least number of decimal numbers, e.g., sum of three values 35.6, 0.162 and 71.41 should be reported to only to the first decimal place as the value 35.6 is known only to the first decimal place. Thus the answer 107.172 is rounded to 107.2.

Rule 5: In multiplication, retain in each factor the more significant figure than it contain in the factor having the largest uncertainty. The percentage precision of the product cannot be greater than percentage precision of the least precise factor entering into the calculations, e.g., the product of the three figures 0.0121, 25.64 and 1.05782 is 0.0121 × 25.6 × 1.06 = 0.328

Rule 6: In a quotient of experimental members, the final rebuilt has only as many significant figures as the factor with the smallest number of significant figures;

e.g., in the calculation $= \dfrac{(0.0181057)(197.15)(0.218)}{0.4970} = 1.56571$

$= 1.57$

Least number of significant figures is in number 0.218.

Thus, the answer should also be expressed in three significant figures.

Significant figures of some numerical values.

   (i)   100.04   : 5
  (ii) 420×10^{10} : 3
 (iii) 5000×100 : 5
 (iv) 0.02758   : 4
  (v) 0.004   : 1

1.8 Errors: Classification and Minimizations

It is observed that the numerical data obtained in quantitative analysis or determination differ to greater or lesser extent. Sometimes it is difficult to obtain the same measurement when performed under identical conditions. So, the reliability of the results depends upon the magnitude of the difference between the average value and the true value or more probable value. Under such conditions the determination is subjected to *errors*. Error often denotes the estimated uncertainty in a measurement or experiment.

Classification of errors

Errors in any set of measurement can be divided on the basis of determination of magnitude of errors into following categories.

(1) Systematic/determinate or Constant Errors

The determinate errors are the errors that remain in a constant way and to a fixed degree in each of the determinations or affect the series of determination to the same degree. These errors can be avoided and their magnitude can be determined, thereby correcting the measurement.

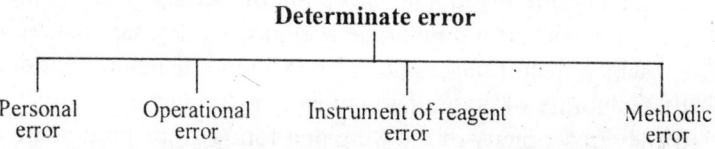

Determinate error

| Personal error | Operational error | Instrument of reagent error | Methodic error |

(i) Personal error: These errors depend on the personal characteristics of an analyst himself. They may arise due to constitutional inability of the individual to make certain observations accurately, e.g.,

    (a) Inability in judging color change sharply in a visual titration which may result in slight overstepping of the end point.

    (b) The estimation of value between two scales division of the burette.

    (c) Inability to detect end point in the titration

    (d) Error in calculations, i.e., induplicate weighing and titration.

    (e) Mechanical loss of material in various steps of analysis during bumping.

(ii) Operational error: These errors are physical in nature and occur when sound analytical technique is not followed. They are easy to detect and eliminate, e.g.,

    (a) Incomplete drying of analytical samples before weighing.

    (b) Under washing of the precipitate which gives consistently excessive results.

(c) Over-washing of the precipitate resulting in systematic losses.

(d) Incorrect draining of the solution from the precipitate.

(iii) Instrument and reagent error: These errors arise from the imperfections in the measuring device and the quality of reagent used, e.g.,

(a) Inequality of the length of the balance arms.

(b) Incorrectly graduated burette.

(c) Using impure reagent.

(d) Incorrect technique involving in the transfer of solutions.

(iv) Methodic errors: These are most serious type of errors encountered in chemical analysis as they are difficult to detect, e.g.,

(a) Differences between the observed end point and the stiochoimetric equivalence point of the reaction.

(b) The main reaction may be accompanied by side reactions which distort the results of the volumetric determination.

(c) Solubility of precipitate in medium and in wash liquid.

(d) Hygroscopicity of the weighing forms of the precipitate.

(e) Volatilization of weighing forms of precipitate on igniting or heating.

(f) The pH meter that has been wrongly standardized.

(g) The indicator used in the reaction may influence the results.

(2) Random or Indeterminate Errors

These errors are indeterminate in magnitude and sign and their appearance does not conform to any laws. Random errors are beyond the control of the observer and are accidental in nature, e.g.,

(i) Fluctuations in temperature and pressure.

(ii) Inability to read marked divisions on a burette or pipette.

(iii) Vibrations in balance during handling.

(iv) Accidental loss of material during analysis.

Indicator error: Due to the logarithmic nature of the pH curve, the transitions are generally extremely sharp, and thus a single drop of titrant just before the endpoint can change the pH significantly, leading to an immediate colour change in the indicator. Therefore, there is a slight difference between the change in indicator color and the actual equivalence point of the titration. This error is referred to as an indicator error, and it is indeterminate.

(3) Errors in Measurement

These errors rise in every measurement, which include any analytical determination, no matter how carefully it is performed. They cannot be prevented or eliminated by correction. However, increasing the number of replicate determinations can considerably reduce them, e.g.,

   (i) Errors in weighing may be due to insensitivity of balance.

  (ii) Wrong suspension of riders.

 (iii) Placing the weights at edge of the pans.

 (iv) Using non-calibrated weights.

(4) Gross Errors

   (i) Use of numerically incorrect inversion factors.

  (ii) Wrong selection of method.

 (iii) Unsuitable storage of samples.

Minimization of Systematic Errors

  (i) *Calibration of apparatus and application of corrections:* For example, periodic calibration of the instrument and apparatus like weights, measuring flasks, pipettes, burettes, and the appropriate correction applied to the original measurements. To reduce systematic errors, recalibrate instruments frequently.

 (ii) *Analysis of standard samples:* This involves carrying out the analysis of a standard sample prepared in such a way that its composition is exactly the same as that of the material to be analyzed.

(iii) *Running a blank determination:* This consists of carrying out a separate determination, the sample being omitted, under exactly the same experimental conditions as are employed in the actual determination of the sample. The object is to find out the effect of the impurities introduced through the reagents and vessels, or to determine the excess of standard solution necessary to establish the end point under the condition met with in the titration of the unknown sample.

(iv) *Use of independent analysis:* In some instances the accuracy of the result may be established by carrying out the analysis in entirely different manner. For example, iron may first be determined gravimetrically as iron (III) oxide. Next it may be determined volumetrically by reducing to the Fe (II) state and titrating with a standard solution of an oxidizing agent, such as $K_2Cr_2O_7$ or Ce (IV) sulphate. In water hardness, the calcium and magnesium concentration determined by atomic absorption may be compared with the results obtained by EDTA titration.

(v) *Running a control determination:* It is carrying out the determination on a standard substance under conditions as close as possible to the experimental conditions. The quantity of the substance should contain the same weight of the constituent as is present in the unknown sample. The weight of the constituent present in the unknown sample can then be calculated from the relation.

$$\frac{\text{Result in standard}}{\text{Result in unknown}} = \frac{\text{Weight of constituent in standard}}{x}$$

Where x is the weight of the constituent in the unknown sample.

1.9 Sampling: Stages and Safety

In pharmaceutical analysis laboratory, the students are supplied with samples that are ready for drying and weighing or in a solution form ready for the subsequent work. Therefore, one does not have to worry with the operation of sampling. However, one should be concerned about the origin, of the samples and how samples are obtained.

In the analysis one is faced with two types of situation:

(i) Either to determine the composition of the pure substance or,

(ii) To determine the average composition of a mass of material.

Sampling is the process of withdrawing a small portion from a bulk of material, which is truly representative of the whole material. Sampling methodologies are usually of three types:

(i) Where all the materials is analysed.

(ii) Casual or random sampling on an adhoc basis.

(iii) Methods in which portion of material is selected upon the statistically probabilities.

The weighing of samples which are liquids and volatile or hygroscopic in nature is done in a small glass container provided with a stopper called *weighing bottle*. However, solid samples may be weighed on a watch glass or directly in a conical flask to save time for analysis.

Stages of Sampling

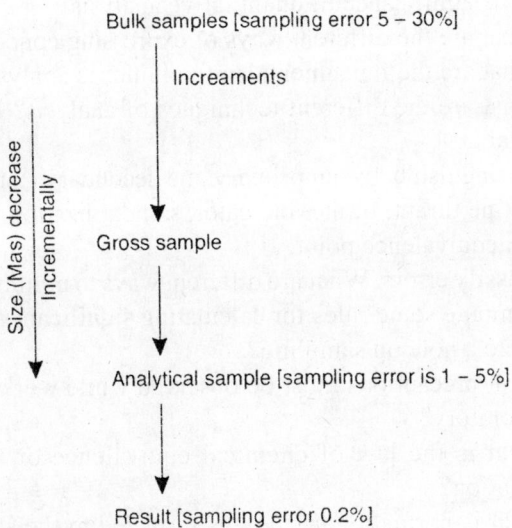

Bulk samples [sampling error 5 – 30%]

Increaments

↓

Gross sample

Size (Mas) decrease

Incrementally

Analytical sample [sampling error is 1 – 5%]

↓

Result [sampling error 0.2%]

Where 'increment' is the successive equal portion of material withdrawn from the bulk sample

Safety During Sampling

(i) The analyst should have good eyesight and must wear the protective clothing and appliances appropriate to the native of hazards.

(ii) He should ensure the proper disposal of used samples.

(iii) Precautions should be taken while handling oils, brushing chemicals and inflammable solvents.

EXERCISES

---

1. What do understand by quantitative analysis? How many types of quantitative chemical analysis are there?
2. Explain different types of volumetric analysis in details with examples.
3. Explain systematic and random error with examples.
4. Distinguish between precision and accuracy.
5. Write a note on significant figures. Discuss zero as significant figure.
6. Give significance of quantitative analysis.
7. What are the different ways of expressing concentration?
8. What are the fundamentals of volumetric analysis?
9. What are the different techniques of analysis? Explain in detail.
10. Distinguish between primary and secondary standard.
11. Define titrant, titrate, indicator, standardization, end point and equivalence point.
12. Classify errors. What are different ways to minimize them?
13. Compute some rules for calculating significant figures.
14. Write a note on sampling?
15. What precautions must be observed while working in the laboratory?
16. What is the law of chemical equivalence or normality equation?
17. What is normality and how is it related to the strength of the solution?
18. What are the requirements that a primary standard should satisfy?

19. What are precision measures? How will calculate mean and standard mean deviation.
20. Give the formula used for calculating the equivalent weights of acid, base and a salt.
21. Write a short note on special techniques in quantitative analysis.
22. What is standard solution? Give method of preparation and classification.

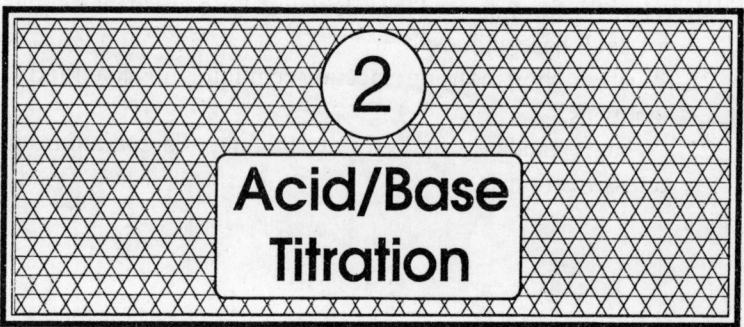

2

Acid/Base Titration

Neutralization or acid/base titrations in pharmaceutical analysis allow quantitative analysis of concentration of an unknown acid or base solution. It makes use of the neutralization reaction, which is the reaction between an acid and a base, producing a salt and water. For example reaction between hydrochloric acid and sodium hydroxide form sodium chloride and water.

$$HCl + NaOH \longrightarrow NaCl + H_2O$$
Hydrochloric acid   Sodium chloride

A volumetric analysis in which a volume of a sample solution is determined by titrating it against standard acid or base using acid-base indicators is also known as **Acid-base titration**. Neutralization is the basis of titration, where a pH indicator shows equivalence point when the equivalent number of moles of a base have been added to an acid.

2.1 Types of Acid/Base Titrations

1. Acidimetry titration: It is a direct or residual volumetric analysis of a base with a standard acid. It is further divided in two parts:

(i) **Direct titration:** It is performed by introducing a standard acid solution gradually from a burette into a solution of base being assayed till the end point is obtained, e.g. assay of sodium bicarbonate.

$$2\,NaHCO_3 + H_2SO_4 \longrightarrow Na_2SO_4 + 2H_2O + 2CO_2$$
Sodium bicarbonate   Sodium sulphate

(ii) Residual titration is used when the rate of reaction between basic compounds with an acid is slow. In this, the solution of the base is treated with an excess of accurately measured standard acid and the excess acid is subsequently titrated with standard base, e.g., assay of zinc oxide.

$$ZnO + H_2SO_4 \longrightarrow ZnSO_4 + H_2O$$
Zinc oxide   Zinc sulphate

2. Alkalimetry titration: It is estimation of acid/acidic drugs by titration with standard alkali. It is further divided in two parts:

(i) Direct titration: It is performed by introducing a standard base solution gradually from a burette into a solution of acid being assayed till the end point is obtained, e.g., assay of boric acid (H_3BO_3). (Fig. 2.1)

$$H_3BO_3 + 2NaOH \longrightarrow Na_2BO_4 + 2H_2O$$
Boric acid   Sodium borate

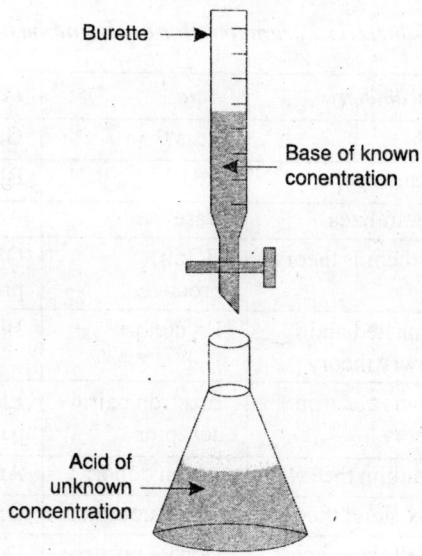

Burette

Base of known conentration

Acid of unknown concentration

Fig.2.1: *Direct titration in alkalimetry*

(ii) **Residual titration:** It is used when the rate of reaction between acidic compounds with a base is slow. In this the solution of the acid is treated with an excess of accurately measured standard base and the excess base is subsequently titrated with standard acid, e.g., assay of aspirin.

Important Definitions of Acid and Base

Acid

(1) A substance with combines with an alkali or a base to form a salt.

(2) A substance or solution which turns blue litmus paper into red.

(3) A solution having pH less than 7.

Base

(1) An electropositive element or radical that combines with an acid to from a salt.

(2) A substance or solution which turns red litmus paper into blue.

(3) A solution having pH greater than 7.

More precisely the acid and base are defined by including parameters given in Table 2.1.

Table.2.1: Parameters for acids and bases

S. No.	Parameter	Acid	Base
1	pH	Less than 7	Greater than 7
2	Litmus paper	Red	Blue
3	Neutralizes	Base	Acid
4	Arrhenius theory	$H^+(aq)$ producer	OH^- (aq) producer
5	Bronsted and Lowry theory	H^+ donor	H^+ acceptor
6	Lewis electron theory	Electron pair acceptor	Electron pair donor
7	Franklin theory	Anion donor	Anion acceptor
8	Lux flood theory	Oxide acceptor	Oxide donor
9	The Usanovich definition	Donate positive ions	Donate negative ions

2.2 Concepts/Theories of Acid and Base Titrations

1. Classic Concept or Arrhenius Concept

The Arrhenius definition of acid-base reactions was devised by **Svante Arrhenius** in 1887 which depends upon the ionization of acids and bases in water.

According to him, "an acid is a substance which when dissolved in H_2O undergoes dissociation with the formation of hydrogen ion $H^+_{(aq)}$ or $H_3O^+_{(aq)}$ and a base is a substance which when dissolved in H_2O undergoes dissociation with the formation of hydroxyl ion $OH^-_{(aq)}$."

$$\text{(Acid) HA} \longrightarrow H^+_{(aq)} + A^-$$

$$\text{(Base) BOH} \longrightarrow B^+ + OH^-_{(aq)}$$

$$HCl \rightleftharpoons H^+ + Cl^- \text{ and } NaOH \rightleftharpoons Na^+ + OH^-$$

$$CH_3COOH \rightleftharpoons H^+ + CH_3COO^- \text{ and}$$

$$NH_4OH \rightleftharpoons NH_4^+ + OH^-$$

The properties of an acid are due to H^+ ions and that of base are due to OH^- ions.

Limitations

(i) The proton or hydrogen ion (H^+) does not exist in an unhydrate form in aqueous solution hence combines with another molecule of H_2O to form $H_3O^+_{(aq)}$ ions.

(ii) It could not explain the basic nature of substance like NH_3 and Na_2CO_3 which do not contain OH^- ions.

(iii) It could not explain the acidic nature of O_2 and SO_2 which do not contain H^+ ions.

(iv) Theory is not applicable to solid substance because dissociation in H_2O is must.

(v) This theory explains the quantitative acid-base behavior in aqueous solution but does not account for acid base behavior in non-aqueous solvents.

2. Bronsted (Danish) and Lowry (British) Concept

The Bronsted-Lowry definition, formulated independently by its two proponents **Johannes Nicolaus Bronsted** and **Martin Lowry** in 1923 is based upon the idea of protonation of bases through the de-protonation of acids, more commonly referred to as the ability of acids to donate hydrogen ions (H^+) or protons to bases, which accept them. According to Bronsted and Lowry concept, 'an acid is a substance that tends to lose protons or an a base in a proton donor while a base is a substance that tends to gain proton or a base is a proton acceptor'. According to this definition acids and bases are related as;

$$A \longrightarrow H^+ + B$$

Acid   Proton   Base

The acid A, and base B are said to form a 'conjugate pair'.

Conjugate pairs: A pair of substance which can be formed from one another by the gain or lose of proton are called as conjugate pairs. If the pairing is between acid and base, it is known as **acid-base conjugate pairs**. Every acid has its conjugate base and every base has its conjugate acid. In a given acid-base conjugate pair; at least one member is an ion, e.g;

(i) $HCl \rightleftharpoons H^+ + Cl^-$

      (Acid)   (Proton)   (Conjugate base)

(ii) $NH_4^+ \rightleftharpoons NH_3 + H^+$

      (Acid)   (Conjugate base)   (Proton)

(iii) $H_3PO_4 \rightleftharpoons H^+ + H_2PO_4^-$

   (Phosphoric   (Proton)   (Conjugate base)
   acid)

(iv) $CH_3 COOH$ (Acid)

$$\updownarrow$$

$$H^+ + CH_3COO^-$$

Proton   Conjugate Base

A conjugate base could be electrically neutral, e.g., NH_3 or a negative ion as $H_2PO_4^-$

(a) $NH_3 + H^+ \rightleftharpoons NH_4^+$

(b) $SO_4^{2-} + H^+ \rightleftharpoons HSO_4^- + H^+ \rightleftharpoons H_2SO_4$ [Acid]

(c) $H_2PO_4^- + H^+ \rightleftharpoons H_3PO_4$

    (Base)   (Proton)   (Conjugate base)

To express the relationship between conjugate acid/base pairs, the following relationship is used:

$$Acid_1 + Base_2 \rightleftharpoons Acid_2 + Base_1$$

Where $Base_1$: Conjugate base of $Acid_1$.

      $Acid_2$: Conjugate acid of $Base_2$.

For example;

$$Acid_1 + Base_2 \rightleftharpoons Acid_2 + Base_1$$

$$HCl + H_2O \rightleftharpoons H_3O^+ + Cl^-$$

$$H_3PO_4 + H_2O \rightleftharpoons H_3O^+ + H_2PO_4^-$$

$$NH_4^+ + H_2O \rightleftharpoons H_3O^+ + NH_3$$

$$HNO_3 + NH_3 \rightleftharpoons NH_4^+ + NO_3^-$$

Since the acids HNO_3, HCl and HBr are stronger acids than H_3O^+, thus forward reaction are almost complete, according to the Bronsted Lowry concept. Thus, we see in water, the acids like HNO_3, HCl and HBr show equal strength. This is due to the fact that H_2O acts as a base, strong enough to dissociate the above acids to the completion. Hence, water is called levelling agent because it levels them to the same strength and the phenomenon is called **levelling effect of H_2O.**

However, if we take the weaker base than water like CH_3COOH, the dissociation of all the acids will not be completed to such extent. Hence, the dissociation of all the acids will not be completed to the same extent, and the strength of the acids will be differentiated. Thus, CH_3COOH acts as differentiating agent and the phenomenon is called **differentiating effect of CH_3COOH.**

Table.2.2: *Some common conjugate acids and bases in order of their relative strength*

	Conjugate acids	Conjugate bases	
Strongest			Weakest
	$HClO_4$	ClO_4^-	
	H_2SO_4	HSO_4^-	
	HCl	Cl^-	
Strength increasing	H_3O^+	H_2O	Strength increasing
	HSO_4^-	SO_4^{2-}	
	HF	F^-	
	CH_3COOH	CH_3COO^-	
	H_2S	HS^-	
	NH_4^+	NH_3	
	HCO_3^-	CO_3^{2-}	
	H_2O	OH^-	
	HS^-	S^{2-}	
	OH^-	O^{2-}	
Weakest			Strongest

Conclusions Drawn from Bronsted Lowry Concept of Acids and Bases

1. The presence of solvent is essential for a substance to act as an acid or a base, e.g., (dry HCl does not turn blue litmus red).

$$HCl + H_2O \longrightarrow H_3O^+ + Cl^-$$

2. A substance is able to show its acidic character only if another substance capable of accepting proton is present. (HCl don't show acidic nature in benzene).

3. Ions may also act as acids or bases.

$$\underset{\text{(Base)}}{Cl^-} + \underset{\text{(Acid)}}{H_3O^+} \longrightarrow \underset{\text{(Acid)}}{HCl} + \underset{\text{(Base)}}{H_2O}$$

Monoprotic acid: It is an acid which gives only one proton on dissociation, e.g., HCl, HNO_3 and CH_3COOH. The boric acid

(H_3BO_3) is a monoprotic acid and weak Lewis acid as it furnishes only one proton on hydrolysis as;

$$H_3BO_3 + H_2O \longrightarrow H^+ + B(OH)_4^-$$

Diprotic acid: It is an acid which dissociates to give one more proton in succession, e.g., H_2SO_4, H_2CO_3 (carbonic acid)

$$H_2SO_4 + H_2O \rightleftharpoons H_3O^+ + HSO_4^-$$

$$\Updownarrow$$

$$SO_4^{2-} + H^+$$

Triprotic acid: It is an acid which furnishes three types of anions. For example, H_3PO_4 furnishes $H_2PO_4^-$, HPO_4^{2-} and PO_4^{3-}.

Monoprotic bases: These can accept one proton

$$HS^- + H^+ \rightleftharpoons H_2S$$

$$H_2O + H^+ \rightleftharpoons H_3O^+$$

Polyprotic bases: These can accept two or more protons, e.g.;

$$SO_4^{2-} + 2H^+ \rightleftharpoons H_2SO_4 \text{ (Sulphuric acid)}$$

$$PO_4^{3-} + 3H^+ \rightleftharpoons H_3PO_4 \text{ (Phosphoric acid)}$$

Amphiprotic substance: Molecules or ions that can behave both as bronsted acids and bases are called amphiprotic substances. Examples are H_2O and HCO_3^-.

With HCl, water acts as a base in accepting a proton from the acid,

$$\underset{\text{(Acid)}}{HCl} + \underset{\text{(Base)}}{H_2O} \rightleftharpoons H_3O^+ + Cl^-$$

However, water is an acid donating a proton to NH_3

$$\underset{\text{(Base)}}{NH_3} + \underset{\text{(Acid)}}{H_2O} \rightleftharpoons NH_4^+ + OH^-$$

The strongest acid has higher tendency to denote proton and will always produce weak conjugate base and weak acid will produce strong conjugate base and vice versa.

$$\underset{\text{(Strong acid)}}{HCl} + H_2O \rightleftharpoons H_3O^+ + \underset{\text{(Weak conjugate base)}}{Cl^-}$$

$$\underset{\text{(Weak acid)}}{CH_3COOH} + \underset{\text{(Base)}}{H_2O} \rightleftharpoons \underset{\text{(Acid)}}{H_3O^+} + \underset{\text{(Strong conjugate base)}}{CH_3COO^-}$$

Same is the case with strong and weak bases as:

$$NH_3 \; + \; H_2O \; \rightleftharpoons \; NH_4^+ \; + \; OH^-$$

(Base)   (Acid)   (Weak conjugate acid)

HCO^-_3 can act as both Bronsted acid and base because it can donate a proton to form CO^{2-}_3 and it can accept the proton to yeild H_2CO_3.

Limitations

1. Behaviors of SO_2, SO_3 and CO_2 as acids and behavior of CaO and BaO_2 as bases.

2. Donating and accepting a proton is must for showing acidic behavior.

3. Acid/base behavior depends upon the presence or absence of solvent.

4. It cannot explain the acid-base reaction taking place in non-protic solvents, like BrF_3, $AlCl_3$ and $POCl_3$ in which no transfer of protons take place.

3. Lewis Theory: [Electronic Theory] (1923)

The Lewis definition of acid base reactions, devised by **Gilbert N. Lewis** in 1923, is an encompassing theory to the Bronsted/Lowry and solvent-system definitions. It is based on a donation mechanism, which conversely attributes the donation and acceptance of electron pairs from bases and acceptance from acids, rather than protons or other bonded substances and spans both aqueous and non-aqueous reactions.

According to him, "An acid is a substance which can accept a pair of electrons to form a coordinate covalent bond, whereas as base is a substance which can donate a pair of electrons to form a coordinate covalent bond. In other words, an acid is an electron acceptor and a base is an electron donor, e.g.,

Lewis acids are $AlCl_3$, $ZnCl_2$, $FeCl_2$, SO_3, SO_2 and $(CH_3)_3$ Br.

Lewis bases are NH_3, $CH_3 - O - CH_3$, CH_2OH, CaO, and H_2O.

The reaction between SO_3 and CaO to form $CaSO_4$ can be represented as follows;

$$CaO \quad + \quad SO_3 \quad \rightleftharpoons \quad CaSO_4$$

Calcium oxide	Sulphure trioxide	Calcium Sulphate
acid	acid	salt

BF_3 accepts a pair of electrons from NH_3 hence, BF_3 is a Lewis acid and NH_3 is a Lewis base. The reaction of boronitriflouride (acid) with ammonia (base) results into a stable octet configuration between mutual sharing of a pair of electrons of the later (donor) and former (acceptor).

Limitation: The relative strength of acids and bases cannot be explained by this concept.

Table 2.3: *Three models of acids and bases*

Model/concept	Definition of acid	Definition of base
Arrhenius (1887)	H^+ producer	OH^- producer
Bronsted–Lowry (1923)	H^+ donor	H^+ acceptor
G. N. Lewis (1939)	Electron – pair acceptor	Electron–pair donor

Note: All Arrhenius acids are also Bronsted acids but all Arrhenius bases are not Bronsted bases. Similarly, all Bronsted bases are Lewis bases but all Bronsted acids are not Lewis acids.

4. Lux–Flood Concept

This concept for acids and bases was firstly proposed by Lux and was extended by Flood, hence called Lux-flood concept of acids and bases. According to this concept, an acid is a substance which accept oxide ion while a base is a substance which donates oxide ion. In other words, acids act as oxide receptors while bases as oxide donors, e.g.,

$$CaO + SiO_2 \longrightarrow CaSiO_3$$

(Base)	(Acid)	(Salt)

In this case, SiO_2 is accepting the oxide ion; hence acting as an acid while CaO is donating the oxide ion, hence acting as a base.

$$\underset{\text{(Base)}}{BaO} + \underset{\text{(Acid)}}{CO_2} \longrightarrow BaCO_3$$

$$\underset{\text{(Base)}}{6\,Na2} + \underset{\text{(Acid)}}{P_4O_{10}} \longrightarrow 4\,Na_3PO_4$$

$$\underset{\text{(Base)}}{NO_3^-} + \underset{\text{(Acid)}}{S_2O_7^{2-}} \longrightarrow NO_2^+ + 2\,SO_4^{2-}$$

Limitations: This concept involves only acids and bases containing oxide ions.

5. Franklin/Solvent System Concept

This definition is based on a generalization of the earlier Arrhenius definition to all auto dissociating solvents. In all such solvents there is a certain concentration of a positive species, **solvonium cations** and negative species, **solvate anions**, in equilibrium with the neutral solvent molecules.

According to **Franklin**, "an acid is a substance which gives rise to a cation, characteristic of respective solvent" and "base is a substance which gives rise to a an anion, characteristics of respective solvent."

$$\underset{\text{(Acid)}}{2\,H_2O} \rightleftharpoons H_3O^+ \text{ (Hydronium)} + OH^- \text{ (Hydroxide)}$$

$$\underset{\text{(Base)}}{2\,NH_3} \rightleftharpoons NH_4^+ \text{ (Ammonium)} + NH_2^- \text{ (Amide)}$$

A solute causing an increase in the concentration of the solvonium ions and a decrease in solvate ions is an acid and one causing the reverse is a base. Thus, in liquid ammonia, NH_3 (supplying NH_2^-) is a strong base.

Self-ionization of water: The self-ionization of water is the chemical reaction in which two water molecules react to produce a hydronium (H_3O^+) and a hydroxide ion (OH^-):

$$2\,H_2O \text{ (l)} \rightleftharpoons H_3O^+ \text{ (aq)} + OH^- \text{ (aq)}$$

The reaction is also known as the auto-ionization or auto dissociation of water. It is an example of autoprotolysis, and relies on the amphoteric nature of water. Water, however pure, is not a simple collection of H_2O molecules. Even in "pure" water, sensitive equipment can detect a very slight electrical conductivity of

0.055 µS. According to the theory of Svante Arrhenius, this must be due to the presence of ions.

Concentration and Frequency

The preceding reaction has a chemical equilibrium constant of $K_{eq} = ([H_3O^+][OH^-]) / [H_2O] = 1.8 \times 10^{-16}$. For reactions in water (or any aqueous solutions), the molarity (a unit of concentration) of water, $[H_2O]$, is practically constant and is omitted from the equilibrium constant expression by convention. The resulting equilibrium constant is called the **ionization constant**, dissociation constant, or self-ionization constant, or ionic product of water and is symbolized by K_w.

$$K_w = K_{eq}[H_2O] = [H_3O^+][OH^-]$$

Where $[H_3O^+]$ = molar concentration of hydrogen or hydronium ion, and

   $[OH^-]$ = molar concentration of hydroxide ion.

The solvent ionizes in the solution by itself to give its characteristic ions. Hence this concept is also called auto-ionization concept, e.g,

H_2O: Water ionizes as

$$2H_2O \rightleftharpoons H_3O^+ + OH^-$$

Acid ion   Base ion

It means that substances which give H_3O^+ are acids while which give OH^- are bases.

e.g., $HCl + H_2O \rightleftharpoons H_3O^+ + Cl^-$

(Solvent cation of H_2O)

$$NH_3 + H_2O \rightleftharpoons NH_4^+ + OH^-$$

(Solvent anion of H_2O)

$$H^+ + OH^-$$

Hence H_2O behaves as an acid and a base, respectively.

Limitations: It considers only the chemical properties of the solvent and ignores the physical properties.

6. The Usanovich Definition

The most general definition is that of the Russian chemist **Mikhail Usanovich**, and can basically be summarized as, an acid as anything that accepts negative species or donates positive ions, and a base as the reverse. The Usanovich concept in a much broader sense includes all the oxidizing agents as acids and the reducing agents as bases, e.g.,

$$Fe^{2+} \longrightarrow Fe^{3+} + e^-$$

(Base)   (Acid)

In the Fe^{3+}/Fe^{2+} systems, the ferric ion (III) acts as an oxidizing agent and is an acid; while the ferrous ion (II) acts as a reducing agent and is a base.

7. The Pearson Definition

In 1963, **Ralph Pearson** proposed an advanced qualitative concept known as Hard Soft Acid Base principle, later made quantitative with help of Robert Parr in 1984. According to this theory alkali metal ions or other light metals with no or few d-electrons or metal ions in higher oxidation states are classified as **hard acids**. Such acids are small in size and their electron charge cloud is not easily polarizable. On the other hand heavier metal ions with nearly complete d-shell are classified as **soft acids**.

Ligands which choose to form most stable complexes with hard acids are classed as **hard bases,** and those which choose to form most stable complexes with soft acids are classed as **soft bases.** The hard bases are anions such as NH_3, H_2O, N_2H_4, and are not easily polarizable. Similarly soft bases are easily polarizable like CN^-, I^-, C_6H_6 and CO.

2.3 Law of Mass Action

This law was first of all interpreted by Guldberg and Wage in 1897 and it stated as; "the rate of chemical reactions is directly proportional to the product of 'active masses 'of the reactants". The term active masses represents the 'molar concentrations' and expressed as moles/liter.

Let us consider a following reversible reaction in moles per liter.

$$[A] + [B] \rightleftharpoons [C] + [D]$$

The square [ ] bracket indicates the concentration of respective components.

According to law of mass action:

Rate of forward reaction $(R_f) \propto [A] \times [B]$, similarly

Rate of Reverse reaction $(R_r) \propto [C] \times [D]$

or $\qquad R_f \propto [A][B] \qquad$ and $\quad R_r \propto [C][D]$

or $\qquad R_f = K_f [A][B]$ and $\quad R_r = K_r [C][D]$

Where K_f and K_r are the proportionately constant for forward and reverse reactions respectively. At equilibrium (concentration at both sides are equal)

or $\qquad \dfrac{K_f}{K_r} = \dfrac{[C].[D]}{[A].[B]}$

or $\qquad K = \dfrac{[C].[D]}{[A].[B]}$ $\qquad\qquad$ ...(i)

Where $K = \dfrac{K_f}{K_r}$ and is called the **'Equilibrium constant'** of the reaction and the equation (i) represent the law of chemical equilibrium.

Application of Law of mass action

Dissociation of H_2O

$$\underset{K_f}{H_2O} \rightleftharpoons \underset{K_r}{H^+ + OH^-}$$

According to law of mass action;

$$K = \dfrac{\left[H^+\right] + \left[OH^-\right]}{[H_2O]}$$

In case of pure H_2O and dilute aqueous solution the concentration of free H_2O may be considered constant because it is slightly ionized and hence, and activity of unionized water molecules is taken as unity.

$$K_W = [\text{H}^+][\text{OH}^-]$$

K_W = Ionic product of H_2O or ionization constants of H_2O and its value is equal to 1×10^{-14}.

2.4 Hydrogen Ion Concentration (pH)

The concept of pH was first introduced by Danish chemist **S. P. L. Sorensen** in 1909. The hydrogen ion concentration or pH is defined as negative logarithm (to base 10) of the concentration of H^+ ion in solution.

However, pH is actually an expression for its mathematical approximation in chemistry. A small *p* is used in place of writing $\log_{10}$ and the H should more correctly be $[\text{H}^+]$, standing for concentration of hydrogen ions.

The formula for calculating pH is:

$$pH = -\log_{10} \alpha_{\text{H}}^+$$

Where α_{H}^+ denotes the activity of H^+ ions, and is dimensionless.

or $\qquad pH = -\log_{10}[\text{H}^+]$

or $\qquad pH = -\log[\text{H}^+]$

$$= \log \frac{1}{\left[\text{H}^+\right]}$$

Applying ($\log m/n = \log m - \log n$) we get,

$$pH = \log[1] - \log[\text{H}^+]$$
$$pH = 0 - \log[\text{H}^+]$$
$$pH = -\log[\text{H}^+] \text{ (Equation derived)}$$

Hydroxyl Ion Concentration (pOH)

There is also pOH, in a sense the opposite of pH, which measures the concentration of OH^- ions, or the basicity of the solution. Since water self ionizes, and notating $[\text{OH}^-]$ as the concentration of hydroxide ions, we have

$$K_w = \alpha_{\text{H}}^+ + \alpha_{\text{OH}}^- = 10^{-14}$$

Where K_w is the ionization constant or ionic product of the water.

pH scale: The pH is defined as,

$$pH = -\log_{10}[H^+]$$

All degrees of acidity and alkalinity between that of solution molar or normal with respect to hydrogen and hydroxyl ions can be expressed by a series of positive numbers between 0 and 14 in a pH scale or can be expressed quantitatively by hydrogen ion concentration. In neutral solution $[H^+] = [OH^-] = 10^{-7}$.

The relationship between $[H^+]$ and pH is shown on the **scale** called pH scale given below:

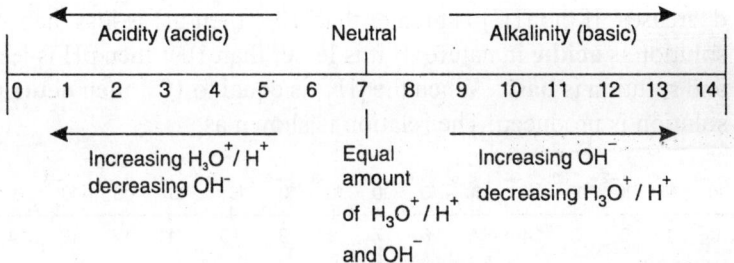

Fig. 2.2: The pH scale

Table. 2.4: *Acidic and alkaline solution with their pH valves.*

$[H^+]$	pH value	$[H^+]$	pH value
10^{-0}	0	10^{-8}	8
10^{-1}	1	10^{-9}	9
10^{-2}	2	10^{-10}	10
10^{-3}	3	10^{-11}	11
10^{-4}	4	10^{-12}	12
10^{-5}	5	10^{-13}	13
10^{-6}	6	10^{-14}	14

$$\begin{aligned}
\text{In acidic solution} \quad &\rightarrow \quad [H^+] > 10^{-7} \\
\text{In alkaline solution} \quad &\rightarrow \quad [H^+] < 10^{-7} \text{ and} \\
\text{In neutral solution} \quad &\rightarrow \quad [H^+] = 10^{-7}
\end{aligned}$$

At pH = 7.0, $[H^+] = [OH^-]$, and the aqueous solution is said to be neutral. The pH values less than 7.0 are acidic, while those with a pH value greater than 7.0 are alkaline or basic. Note that theoretically, pH values may be less than 0 or greater than 14. Concentrated hydrochloric acid is about 10 mol.dm^{-3}. If it was completely dissociated at that concentration, it would give a hydrogen ion concentration, [H$^+$] of 10, corresponding to a pH = –1.

Since we know that pH = log $\dfrac{1}{\left[H^+\right]}$ or pH ∝ $\dfrac{1}{\left[H^+\right]}$, i.e., pH is

inversely proportional to H$^+$ concentration. Therefore, if the [H$^+$] increases, the hydrogen ion concentration or pH of solution decreases. If the [H$^+$] is greater than 10^{-7} then pH is less, hence, solution is **acidic** in nature. If it is lesser than 10^{-7} then pH is less and solution is **basic**. When the [H$^+$] is equal to 10^{-7} then **neutral** solution is produced. The relation is shown as;

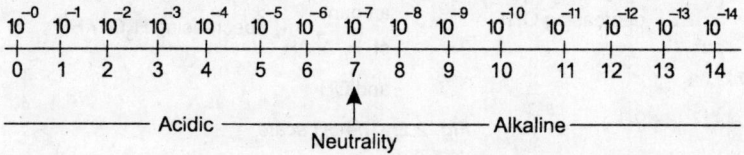

Fig. 2.3: *Relation between H$^+$ concentration and pH valve*

Equation of pH for pure H$_2$O

$$K_W = 1 \times 10^{-14} \text{ (Ionic product of water)}$$
$$[H^+] = 10^{-7}$$
$$[OH^-] = 10^{-7}$$

It means that in pure water the concentration of H$^+$ and OH$^-$ ions is 10^{-7} g ion per liter each.

$$pH = -\log[H^+]$$
$$pH = -\log[10^{-7}]$$
$$= -\log[1/10^7]$$
$$= -[\log 1 - \log 10^7]$$
$$= -[0 - \log 10^7]$$
$$pH = 0 + \log 10^7$$
$$pH = 7 \log 10$$
$$pH = 7 \times 1 = 7 \text{ (Neutral pH for H}_2\text{O molecule)}.$$

Applications: The application of pH in pharmacy is given as;

(i) According to IP, human insulin is maintained at pH 3.0–3.5 by adding HCl.

(ii) Lowering the pH of antiseptic creams and solutions increases their antimicrobial activity.

(iii) In slightly soluble acid drugs e.g.

    (a) Acetyl salicylic acid

    (b) Theophyline

    (c) Sulphonamide

(iv) The stability of following drugs is increased in acidic medium;

    (a) Adrenaline: 3.2–3.6

    (b) Ergotamine: 3.3

(v) Absorption of drugs upon pH of the physiological fluid, e.g., use of intravenous injection should be buffered to pH of about 7.35.

(vi) In acidic pH the drugs can be preserved for longer periods, i.e., their shelf life can be increased.

pH of 0.1 m HCl

$$HCl \rightleftharpoons H^+ + Cl^-$$

The HCl is completely dissociated into the $[H^+]$ ions, therefore

$$HCl = [H^+]$$
$$[0.1\ m] = [0.1\ m]$$
$$= 10^{-1}\ \text{ions/litre}$$
$$\therefore \quad pH = -\log[H^+]$$
$$= -\log[10^{-1}]$$
$$= -\log[1/10] \quad [\text{Applying } \log m/n = \log m - \log n]$$
$$pH = 1$$

Hence, pH of the 0.1 N HCl is found out to be 1

pH for 2 g of NaOH in 1 litre of solution

Weight of NaOH taken = 2 g

Volume = 1 litre

$$\text{Molarity} = \frac{n(moles)}{v(voles)} = \frac{Wt/mol.wt\ o\ f\ n\ NaOH}{V}$$

$$= \frac{2/40}{1}$$

$$= 0.05 \text{ M [Molecular wt of NaOH = 40]}$$

$[H^+]$ can be calculated as:

$$[H^+] = \frac{K_W}{\left[OH^-\right]} = \frac{1 \times 10^{-14}}{0.05} = 2 \times 10^{-13}$$

Since $pH = -\log [H^+]$ [or]

∴ $pH = -\log[2 \times 10^{-3}]$

            $= -[\log 2 + \log 10^{-13}]$

            $= -(0.3010 - 13)$

       $pH = +12.699$

The pH of the NaOH solution is found to be **12.699.**

2.5 Common Ion Effect

The **common-ion effect** is an application of Le-Chateliers principle (1884) which states as: "if a change in concentration is caused to a chemical reaction in equilibrium, the equilibrium will shift to the right or left so as to minimize or reduce the change that has occurred".

The common-ion effect is also defined in following ways;

1. The reduction or repression of the degree of ionization or dissociation of an acid or salt by addition of common ion.
2. The effect on a solution of two dissolved solutes that contain the same ion.
3. When a solution has an ion introduced from another source that is the same as one of the ions in the original solution, the effect predicted by Le-Chateliers principle is called the common ion effect. The presence of a common ion suppresses the ionization of a weak acid or a weak base.

When a soluble salt (say AC) is added to a solution of another salt (AB) containing a common ion A^+, the dissociation of AB is suppressed according to the Le-Chateliers principle as equilibrium will shift to the left thereby decreasing the concentration of A^+. The dissociation is shown as;

$$[AB] \rightleftharpoons [A^+] + [B^+]$$

$$[AC] \rightleftharpoons [A^+] + [C^+]$$

Therefore, due to common ion effect the degree of dissociation of the AB will be reduced, e.g., if sodium acetate and acetic acid are dissolved in the same solution, they both dissociate and ionize to produce acetate ions. Sodium acetate is a strong electrolyte so it dissociates completely in solution. Acetic acid is a weak acid so it ionizes slightly in the solution as;

$$CH_3COOH_{(l)} \rightleftharpoons H^+_{(aq)} + CH_3COO^-_{(aq)}$$

$$CH_3COONa_{(s)} \longrightarrow Na_{(aq)} + CH_3COO^-_{(aq)}$$

According to Le-Chateliers principle, the addition of acetate ions as common ion from sodium acetate will suppress the ionization of acetic acid and shifts its equilibrium to the left. Thus, the dissociation of the acetic acid will decrease and the pH of the solution will increase. This will decrease the hydrogen ion concentration as pH $\propto \dfrac{1}{H^+}$ and thus the common-ion solution

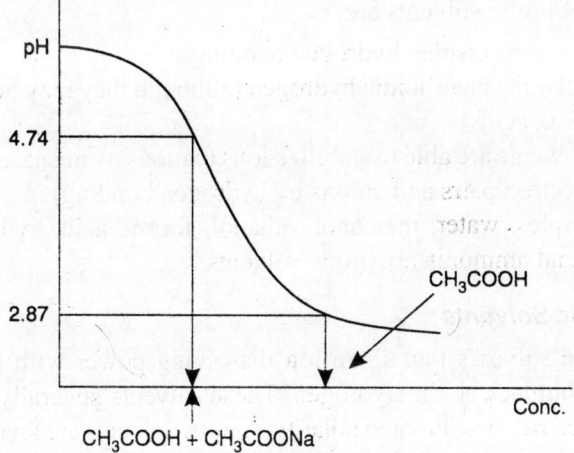

Fig. 2.4: *Common ion effect*

will be less acidic than a solution containing only acetic acid. Therefore, 0.1M acetic acid solution has a pH of 2.87 but a solution of 0.1M acetic acid and 0.1M sodium acetate has a pH of 4.74. The pH of a buffer is 4.74 which is higher than acid itself due to common ion effect.

2.6 Role of Solvents in Acid-Base Titration

The concept of solvents in acid-base titration was discussed by Lowry and Bronsted in auto-protonation or auto-ionization. In acid base titration generally four types of solvents are used;

1. Protic or Protogenic Solvent

It is capable of acting as a proton (hydrogen) donor strongly or weakly acidic (as a bronsted acid). The term is preferred to the synonym "protic" or "acidic". It is also called **HBD** (hydrogen bond donor) solvent.

In chemistry a **protic solvent** is a solvent that carries a hydrogen bond between an oxygen as in a hydroxyl group or a nitrogen as in an amine group. More generally, any molecular solvent which contains dissociable H^+, such as hydrogen fluoride, is called a **protic** or **protogenic solvent**. The molecules of such solvents can donate an H^+ (proton). In chemical reactions the use of polar protic solvents favors the S_N1 reaction mechanism. Common characteristics of protic solvents are:

   (i)   Solvents display hydrogen bonding.
  (ii) Solvents have acidic hydrogen (although they may be very weak acids).
 (iii) Solvents are able to stabilize ions (cations by unshared free electron pairs and anions by hydrogen bonding).

For examples, water, methanol, ethanol, formic acid, hydrogen fluoride and ammonia are protic solvents.

2. Aprotic Solvents

These are solvents that share ion dissolving power with protic solvents but lack acidic hydrogen. These solvents generally have high dielectric constants and polarity. Aprotic solvents are favorable for S_N2 reactions. Apart from solvent effects, polar aprotic solvents may also be essential for reactions which use strong bases, such as reactions involving Grignard reagents or n-butyl lithium. The aprotic solvents are dimethyl sulfoxide, dimethylformamide, and picric acid. The picric acid and HCl forms a colourless solution in benzene which becomes yellow on adding aniline. Picric acid doesn't dissociate in benzene solution and in the presence of base aniline it acts as an acid.

3. Protophillic Solvents

These solvents are basic in character and had a strong tendency to bind with proton of an acid to form solvated proton.

$$HCl + NH_3 \rightleftharpoons [NH_4^+] + [Cl^-]$$

Solvated proton

4. Amphiprotic Solvents

These solvents are both protophyllic and protogenic in nature, e.g., water, acetic acid and alcohols.

Dissociation of acetic acid: It is dissociated in small amount as:

$$CH_3COOH \rightleftharpoons CH_3COO^- + H^+$$

If the strong acid like perchloric acid [$HClO_4$] is added in acetic acid, the acetic acid behaves as an base and combines with protons donated by the perchloric acid to form an 'onium ion' which acts as strongly acidic solution due to donating nature of proton to a base;

$$HClO_4 \rightleftharpoons [ClO_4^-] + [H^+]$$

$$CH_3COOH + H^+ \rightleftharpoons CH_3COOH_2^+$$

(Onium ion)

2.7 Relative Strength of Acids and Bases

A strong acid has a tendency to lose proton readily from its molecule and weak acid loses proton slowly from its molecule. Strength of an acid depends on its capacity to produce protons while as strength of base depends on the concentration of the hydroxyl ion in its aqueous solution. The strong acid produces weak conjugate base and the weak acid has strong conjugate base.

Strong acid		**Weak Base**
HCl	$\rightleftharpoons$	$Cl^- + H^+$
H_2SO_4	$\rightleftharpoons$	$SO_4^{2-} + 2H^+$

Weak acid		**Strong Base**
CH_3COOH	$\rightleftharpoons$	$CH_3COO^- + H^+$
H_2O	$\rightleftharpoons$	$OH^- + H^+$

Strength of acid: The strength of an acid, in comparison to other acids, can be determined without the use of pH calculations by observing the following characteristics:

1. **Electronegativity:** The higher the electronegativity of a conjugate base in the same period, the more acidic it would be.
2. **Atomic size:** The larger the conjugate base in the same group, the more acidic.
3. **Charge:** The closer to neutrality an ion is, the more acidic (neutral molecules can be stripped of protons more easily than ions).
4. **Hydrogen ion concentration:** The strength of acid is related to concentration of H^+ ion which it yields on ionization in a solvent.
5. **Degree of dissociation ($\propto$):** It depends upon the value of the degree of dissociation ($\propto$) at a given concentration. To measure the acid strength, the term **acid dissociation constant (Ka)** or dissociation constant of acid is used.

Acid dissociation constant (Ka) gives the relationship between degree of dissociation ($\propto$) and concentration of that acid.

Consider the equation representing the dissociation of an acid (HA)

$$HA \xrightleftharpoons{H_2O} H^+ + A^-$$

Applying law of mass action to the acid dissociation equilibrium, we can write,

$$K_a = \frac{\left[H^+\right]\left[A^-\right]}{[HA]} \qquad \dots (1)$$

Where K_a = acid dissociation constant.

In dilute solutions of the acid [HA], we can assume that the concentration of [HA] remains nearly constant, therefore, term [HA] is not included in equation (i) so

$$K_a = [H^+] \cdot [A^-] \qquad \ldots(2)$$

Strength of acid is defined as the concentration of H^+ ions in its aqueous solution at a given temperature. From the equation (2), it is clear that concentration of hydrogen (ions) $[H^+]$ depends on the value of K_a. Therefore, the value of K_a for a particular acid is a measure of its acid strength or acidity, e.g., for strong acid, value of K_a is large because it dissociates to large extent. For weak acid, value of K_a is small as it is dissociated to lesser extent. It means that, the value of acid dissociation constant is large for a strong acid, while it is small for a weak acid. Units of K_a = mol/L.

The order of strength of some acids is;

$$HClO_2 > HBr > H_2SO_4 > HCl > HNO_3 > H_3PO_4$$

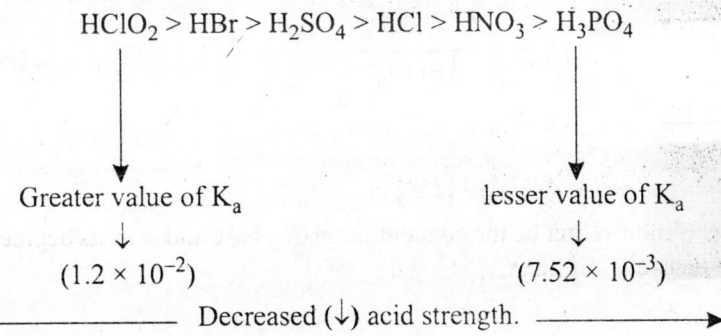

Greater value of K_a lesser value of K_a

(1.2×10^{-2}) (7.52×10^{-3})

———————— Decreased (↓) acid strength. ————→

Relative Strength of Base

According to Arrhenius concept, a base is a substance which in an aqueous solution gives OH^- ions.

Consider a base (BOH) whose dissociation may be represented as;

$$BOH \rightleftharpoons B^+ + OH^-$$

Applying the law of mass action to the above equilibrium, we can write the equilibrium expression as;

$$K_b = \frac{\left[B^+ \right]\left[OH^- \right]}{[BOH]} \qquad \ldots(1)$$

Where K_b is the constant and is called **base dissociation constant**. For dilute solutions of base [BOH], the concentration of BOH remains nearly constant, therefore, term BOH is not included in equation (i) so;

$$K_b = [B^+][OH^-] \qquad ...(2)$$

Thefefore strength of base is defined as 'the concentration of the hydroxyl ion in its aqueous solution at a given temperature'.

From the equation (2) it is clear that the concentration of the hydroxyl ions (OH^-) depends upon the value of K_b. Therefore, the value of K_b for a certain base is a measure of its base strength.

Calculation of K_a or K_b: (Ionization Constant)

The equilibrium expression for the dissociation of a base is given by;

$$K_b = \frac{\left[B^+\right]\left[OH^-\right]}{[BOH]} \qquad ...(a)$$

$$K_a = \frac{\left[H^+\right]\left[A^-\right]}{[HA]}$$

Let C moles/liter be the concentration of a base and $\propto$ as its degree of dissociation, then,

$$K_a = \frac{\left[H^+\right]\left[A^-\right]}{[HA]}$$

$[\overline{A}] = [OH^-] = C\alpha$ and $[H^+] = [B^+] = C\alpha$
$[HA] = [BOH] = C(1-\alpha)$

If 1 mole / litre is concentration, then after dissociation it is equal to $C(1-\alpha)$, substituting these values is the equilibrium expression (a) we have;

$$K_b = \frac{C\alpha \times C\alpha}{C(1-\alpha)}$$

$$K_b = \frac{C^2\alpha^2}{C(1-\alpha)}$$

$$K_b = \frac{C\alpha^2}{(1-\alpha)} \text{ or } K_a = \frac{C\alpha^2}{(1-\alpha)}$$

For weak bases and acids the concentration $(1-\alpha) \cong 1$

Therefore, $K_b = C\alpha^2$ and $K_a = C\alpha^2$

For two different acids and bases, 1 and 2, let the degree of dissociation be α_1 and α_2 dissociation constant K_1 and K_2, Then,

For Acid 1 or Base 1, $\qquad\qquad K_1 = C\alpha_1{}^2$ (i)

For Acid 2 or Base 2, $\qquad\qquad K_2 = C\alpha_2{}^2$ (ii)

Dividing equation (i) by (ii), we have;

$$\frac{K_1}{K_{12}} = \frac{C\alpha_1^2}{C\alpha_2^2} \Rightarrow \frac{\alpha_1}{\alpha_2} = \sqrt{\frac{K_1}{K_2}}$$

Since H^+ is the measure of acid strength and (OH^-) is a measure of base strength and it depends on the degree of dissociation $\propto$, we can write,

$$\frac{\text{Strength of acid or base 1}}{\text{Strength of acid or base 2}} = \sqrt{\frac{K_1}{K_2}}$$

Evidently the ratio $\sqrt{\dfrac{K_1}{K_2}}$ would give us the relative strength of the two acids or bases.

e.g., if $\propto_1$ for formic acid $= 21.4 \times 10^{-5}$ and $\propto_2$ for acetic acid $= 1.81 \times 10^{-5}$.

Then relative strength of the acids is given as:

$$\frac{\text{Strength of HCOOH}}{\text{Strength of CH}_3\text{COOH}} = \sqrt{\frac{K\text{HCOOH}}{K\text{CH}_3\text{COOH}}} = \sqrt{\frac{21.4 \times 10^{-5}}{1.81 \times 10^{-5}}}$$

$$= 3.438:1$$

Therefore, formic acid is 3.438 times stronger than acetic acid.

2.8 Hydrolysis of Salts

Salt: A salt is defined of the chemical substance other than water which is produced by the neutralization of an equivalent amount of

   (i) A strong acid and a strong base.

   (ii) A strong acid and a weak base.

(iii) A weak acid and a strong base and

(iv) A weak acid and a weak base.

Hydrolysis: It is chemical reaction of a compound with water to form new substance.

Salt hydrolysis: The phenomenon in which a salt reacts with water to produce acidic, neutral or alkaline solution is called salt hydrolysis. Or

The reaction in which cation and anion of salt [e.g., NaCl Na$^+$ (cation) and Cl$^-$ (anion)] reacts with H$^+$ and OH$^-$ furnished by water to give acidic, alkaline or neutral solutions is called 'Salt hydrolysis'.

Need of Salt Hydrolysis

1. To check the effect on the concentration of H$^+$ and OH$^-$ during the hydrolysis.

2. To check the nature of the aqueous solution of salt. (e.g., acidic, neutral or basic).

Classifications: On the basis of the nature of their solutions, salts may be of four types:

(i) Salt of Strong Acid and Strong Base

These salts are formed by the reaction of strong acids with strong bases as:

$$HCl + NaOH \rightleftharpoons NaCl + H_2O$$

$$HCl + KOH \rightleftharpoons KCl + H_2O$$

Therefore, for salt hydrolysis:

$$NaCl + H_2O \rightleftharpoons NaOH + HCl$$

$$KCl + H_2O \rightleftharpoons KOH + HCl$$

$$Na_2SO_4 + 2H_2O \rightleftharpoons 2 NaOH + H_2SO_4$$

Salts of strong acids and strong bases do not undergo hydrolysis. Therefore, dissociation of NaCl;

$$NaCl \xrightleftharpoons{H_2O} \underset{\text{Acid}}{Na^+} + \underset{\text{Base}}{Cl^-}$$

In this case, neither the anions have tendency to combine with $[H^+]$ ions nor the cations have tendency to combine with $[OH^-]$ ions. The related acids and bases are strong electrolytes and are completely dissociated. There is no change in concentration of H^+ and OH^- and, therefore, the solution becomes *neutral*.

(ii) Salt of Strong Acid and Weak Base

$$HCl + NH_4OH \rightleftharpoons NH_4Cl + H_2O$$

$$NH_4Cl \rightleftharpoons NH_4^+ + Cl^-$$

Since Cl^- ion does not have tendency to react with $[H^+]$ ions while NH_4^+ (conjugated acid) react with $[OH^-]$ to form undissociated NH_4OH as:

$$NH_4^+ + H_2O \rightleftharpoons NH_4OH + H^+$$
$$\qquad\qquad\qquad\;\; \text{(Weak} \quad \text{(Slightly}$$
$$\qquad\qquad\qquad\;\; \text{base)} \quad \text{dissociating)}$$

Therefore, the aqueous solution of NH_4Cl is always **acidic** in nature due to large concentration of H^+, which returns to the solution.
Salt hydrolysis constant: Hydrolysis of NH_4Cl may be represented as;

$$NH_4Cl + H_2O \rightleftharpoons NH_4OH + H^+$$

$$NH_4^+ + Cl^-$$

or $\qquad NH_4^+ + H_2O \rightleftharpoons NH_4OH + H^+$

Applying law of mass action;

$$K_h = \frac{[NH_4OH].\left[H^+\right]}{\left[NH_4^+\right].[H_2O]}$$

Since for large excess, the water is nearly constant and is equal to unity.

Therefore, $\qquad K_h = \dfrac{[NH_4OH].\left[H^+\right]}{\left[NH_4^+\right]}$

Where K_h = Hydrolysis constant

Relation between K_h, K_w and K_b: $NH_4OH \rightleftharpoons NH_4^+ + H^+$

Applying law of mass action; $K_b = \dfrac{[NH_4][OH^+]}{[NH_4OH]}$ ...(a)

We know $K_W = [H^+][OH^-]$ ...(b)

Dividing (*b*) by (*a*) we have;

$$\frac{K_W}{K_b} = \frac{[H^+].[OH^-]}{[NH_4^+][OH^-]}[NH_4OH] = \frac{[H^+][NH_4OH]}{[NH_4^+]}$$

$$\frac{K_W}{K_b} = K_h \ (\text{as } K_h = \frac{[NH_4OH].[H^+]}{[NH_4^+]})$$

Therefore, weaker the base, greater is hydrolysis constant of salt and, hence, greater the degree of hydrolysis.

In case of reaction between salt of strong acid and strong base, due to strong K_a, the degree of hydrolysis is weaker.

(iii) Salt of Weak Acid and Strong Base

Salt is formed by the action of a weak acid and a strong base, e.g.

$CH_3COOH + NaOH \rightleftharpoons CH_3COONa + H_2O$

$CH_3COONa + H_2O \rightleftharpoons NaOH + CH_3COOH$

    (Strongly   (Weakly
    ionized)   ionized)

$CH_3COO^- + Na^+$

The H^+ are taken by CH_3COO^- leads to increase in the concentration of OH^- and form CH_3COOH, therefore, the solution of this type of salt is **alkaline** in nature due to increased concentration of OH^- ions.

(iv) Salt of Weak Acid and Weak Base

Salt is formed by the action of weak acid and the weak base, e.g.

$CH_3COOH + NH_4OH \rightleftharpoons CH_3COONH_4 + H_2O$

$$CH_3COONH_4 + H_2O \rightleftharpoons NH_4OH + CH_3COOH$$

(Both are weakly ionized)

$$CH_3COO^- + NH_4^+$$

The H^+ and OH^- are equal in concentration; therefore, the solution of this type of salt is **neutral** in nature.

2.9 Buffers, Buffer Solution, Buffer Systems

An electrolyte solution capable of maintaining its pH value relatively constant when either a small acid or base is added is called as buffer solutions. (Or) Solutions of weak acids and salts of their conjugate bases form **buffer solutions**.

Types of Buffers

1. **Acidic buffers**: A buffer of weak acid and its salt, e.g., CH_3COOH and CH_3COONH_4 having pH always less than 7.
2. **Basic buffers**: A buffer of weak base acid and its salt, e.g., NH_4OH and NH_4Cl having pH always greater than 7.

These are the pairs of related chemical compounds. Also in buffer solutions there is a formation of conjugated acid/base pairs.

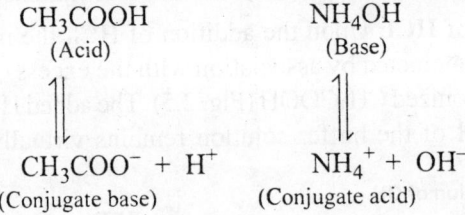

CH_3COOH	NH_4OH
(Acid)	(Base)
$CH_3COO^- + H^+$	$NH_4^+ + OH^-$
(Conjugate base)	(Conjugate acid)

Buffering Agent

Buffering agents can be either the weak acid or weak base that would comprise a buffer solution. Buffering agents are usually added to water to form buffer solutions. They are the substances that are responsible for the buffering action produced in these solutions. These agents are added to substances that are to be placed into acidic or basic conditions in order to stabilize the substance.

For example, buffered aspirin has a buffering agent, such as MgO, that will maintain the pH of the aspirin as it passes through the stomach of the patient. Another use of a buffering agent is in antacid tablets, whose primary purpose is to lower the acidity of the stomach. Buffering agents and buffer solutions are almost one and the same except with few differences.

1. Buffer solutions maintain pH of a system, preventing large changes in it, whereas buffering agents modify the pH.
2. Buffering agents are the active components of buffer solutions.

Monopotassium phosphate (MKP) is an example of a buffering agent. It has a mildly acidic reaction; when applied as a fertilizer with urea or diammonium phosphate, it minimizes pH fluctuations which can cause nitrogen loss.

Regulation of pH in Buffers/Operation of Buffer System

Let us illustrate the buffer action by taking example of common acidic buffer system consisting of a solution of acetic acid and sodium acetate (CH_3COOH/CH_3COONa).

$$CH_3COOH \rightleftharpoons CH_3COO^- + H^+ \qquad ...(1)$$

$$CH_3COONH_4 \rightleftharpoons CH_3COO^- + NH_4^+ \qquad ...(2)$$

Therefore, buffer solution maintains concentration of CH_3COO^- ions produced by complete ionization of sodium acetate.

Addition of HCl: Upon the addition of HCl, the increase of H^+ ions is counteracted by association with the excess of acetate ions to form unionized CH_3COOH (Fig. 2.5). The added H^+ is re-utilized and the pH of the buffer solution remains virtually unchanged.

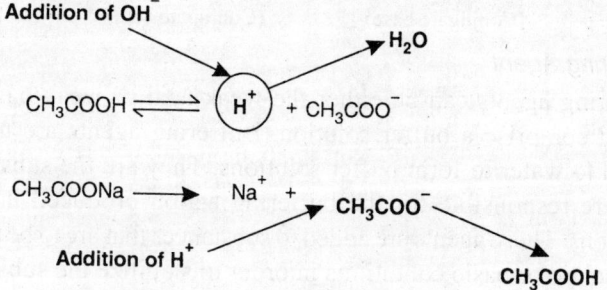

Fig. 2.5: Operation of acidic buffer

However, owing to the increased concentration of CH_3COOH, the equilibrium will shifts slightly to the right to increase H^+ ions. (pH = 4.66). This explains the marginal decrease of pH of the buffer solution on the addition of HCl (Fig. 2.7).

Addition of NaOH: When a sodium hydroxide solution is added to buffer solution, the frequent increase of OH^- ions is counteracted

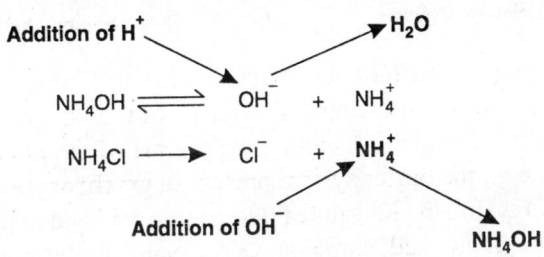

Fig. 2.6: Operation of basic buffer

by association with the excess of ammonium ions to form unionized NH_4OH (Fig. 2.6). The added OH^- is re-utilized and the pH of the buffer solution remains virtually unchanged. Consequently, concentration H^+ is slightly less and pH will be slightly higher than the buffer pH values (pH = 4.83) (Fig. 2.7).

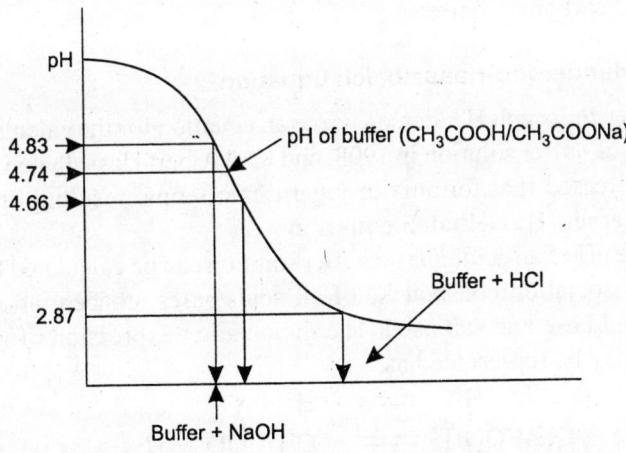

Fig. 2.7: pH of buffer solution on addition of HCl and NaOH

Importance of Different Buffers in Pharmacy

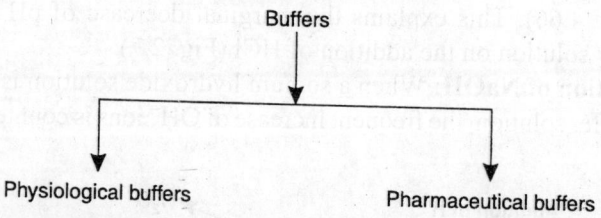

1. Physiological buffers: The physiological or biological buffers are present in the fluid connective tissue of the human body and are usually beneficial in maintaining the pH of the blood almost constant, e.g., the buffer system present in **erythrocyte / RBC** of blood is OxyHb.Hb / K^+ salts of phosphoric acid and in **plasma** of blood is carbonic acid; carbonates / Na^+ salts of phosphoric acid.

2. Pharmaceutical buffers: The buffers used in some pharmaceutical preparations/formulations are given as:

- **Tablets:** $NaHCO_3$, $MgCO_3$, and Na-Citrate buffers.
- **Creams and ointments:** Citric acid and its salts, phosphoric acid and its salts.
- **Parenterals (injections):** Acetate, citrate and glutamate buffers.
- **Ophthalmic (eye) preparations:** Borate, phosphate and carbonate buffers

2.10 Henderson-Hasselbalch Equation

Lawrence Joseph Henderson wrote an equation for the calculation of pH of buffer solution in 1908, and Karl Albert Hasselbalch later re-expressed that formula in logarithmic terms, resulting in the **Henderson-Hasselbalch equation.**

The pH of an acidic/basic buffer solution can be calculated from the dissociation constant K, of all acids/bases, concentration of the acid/base and salt used. The dissociation expression of weak acid may be represented as;

$$HA \rightleftharpoons H^+ + A^-$$
$$CH_3COOH \rightleftharpoons CH_3COO^- + H^+ \quad ...(i)$$
$$CH_3COONH_4 \rightleftharpoons CH_3COO^- + NH_4^+ \quad ...(ii)$$

According to law of mass action:

$$K_a = [H^+] [A^-] / [HA] \text{ or } [H^+] = K_a \frac{[CH_3COOH]}{\left[CH_3COO^-\right]}$$

Where, $[CH_3COOH]$ = representing the total concentration of an acid in solution and
$[CH_3COO^-]$ = representing the total concentration of acetate ion as most of them are entirely contributed by salt (CH_3COONH_4).

$$H^+ = K_a \frac{(\text{Acid})}{(\text{Salt})}$$

Expressing of negative logarithm on both sides we get;

$$-\log [H^+] = -\log K_a - \log \frac{(\text{Acid})}{(\text{Salt})}$$

But $-\log [H^+]$ = pH and
$-\log K_a$ = pK_a

$$pH = pK_a - \log \frac{(\text{Acid})}{(\text{Salt})}$$

$$pH = pK_a + \log \frac{(\text{Salt})}{(\text{Acid})} \quad \text{(Inverting the sign)}$$

This relationship is called Henderson's Hasselbalch equation for acidic buffer. Similarly the Henderson's Hasselbalch equation for a basic buffer can be derived as;

$$pH = pK_b + \log \frac{(\text{Salt})}{(\text{Base})}$$

Significance

1. The pH of the buffer solution can be calculated from the initial concentration of the weak acid and the salt, provided K_a is given.

2. It allows calculation of the ratio in which the weak acid and its salt must be mixed in order to get a buffer solution of known pH.

3. The acid dissociation constant (K_a) can be calculated by measuring the pH of buffer solution containing equimolar concentration of acid / salt.

$$pH = pK_a + \log \frac{(Salt)}{(Base)}$$

$$So \quad pH = pK_a \ as \ \log \frac{(Salt)}{(Base)} = 1$$

The measured pH gives the value of pK_a of the weak acid.

Limitations: There are some significant approximations implicit in the Henderson-Hasselbalch equation. The most significant is the assumption that the concentration of the acid and its conjugate base at equilibrium will remain the same as the formal concentration. This neglects the dissociation of the acid and the hydrolysis of the base. The dissociation of water itself is neglected as well. These approximations will fail when dealing with relatively strong acids or bases.

2.11 The pH Indicator

A pH indicator is a halochromic chemical compound or a compound which changes colour at the change of pH valve. It is added in small amounts to a solution so that the pH (acidity or alkalinity) of the solution can be determined easily. Hence, a pH indicator is a

Bromothymol blue	Y	Y	Y	Y	Y	Y	Y/B	B	B	B	B	B	B	B	B
Litmus	R	R	R	R	R	R/P	P/B	B	B	B	B	B	B	B	B
Methyl orange	Y	Y	Y	Y/R	R	R	R	R	R	R	R	R	R	R	R
Methyl red	Y	Y	Y	Y	Y	Y/R	R	R	R	R	R	R	R	R	R
Phenolphthalein	C	C	C	C	C	C	C	C	C/P	P	P	P	P	P	P
Phenol	Y	Y	Y	Y	Y	Y	Y	Y/R	R	R	R	R	R	R	R
Thymol blue	R	R	R/Y	Y	Y	Y	Y	Y	Y/B	B	B	B	B	B	B

$$0 \quad 1 \quad 2 \quad 3 \quad 4 \quad 5 \quad 6 \quad 7 \quad 8 \quad 9 \quad 10 \quad 11 \quad 12 \quad 13 \quad 14$$

$$\xrightarrow{\hspace{3cm} pH \hspace{3cm}}$$

Where: Y = Yellow; R = Red; B = Blue; P = Pink and C = Colorless

Fig. 2.8: *pH indicators and their colours.*

chemical detector for hydronium ions (H_3O^+) or hydrogen ions (H^+) in the Arrhenius model. Normally, the indicator causes the colour of the solution to change depending on the pH.

Indicators must be carefully chosen so that their colour changes take place at the pH values expected for an aqueous solution of the salt produced in the titration. The commonly used pH indicators are shown in Fig.2.8.The pH indicators themselves are frequently weak acids or bases. When introduced into a solution, they may bind to H^+ (hydrogen ion) or OH^- (hydroxide ion) and different electron configuration of the bound indicator causes the indicator colour to change. Due to subjective determination of colour, pH indicators are susceptible to imprecise readings. For applications requiring precise measurement of pH, a pH meter is frequently used. The pH indicators are frequently employed in titrations in analytical chemistry and biology experiments to determine the extent of a chemical reaction. Indicators usually exhibit intermediate colours at pH values inside the listed transition range. For example, phenol red exhibits an orange colour between pH 6.8 and 8.4 (Table 2.5). The transition range may shift slightly depending on the concentration of the indicator in solution and on the temperature at which it is used. pH values above 7.0 are basic, and pH values below 7.0 are acidic. Solutions with a pH value of 7.0 are neutral. Most pH values range from 1 to 14, but super acids may have a negative pH value. Similarly, super bases may have pH values greater than 14. Natural pH indicators are carrots, cherries, grapes, onion, rhubarb, rose petals and tea.

2.12 Acid-Base Indicators

It is an organic dye that signals the end point of the titration by a visual change in colour according to H^+ concentration. An acid-base indicator is a weak organic acids or bases. The undissociated form of the indicator has a different colour than the ionic form of the indicator. An indicator does not change colour from pure acid to pure alkaline at specific hydrogen ion concentration. The colour change is not sudden and abrupt but occurs over a range of hydrogen ion concentrations (usually about two pH units). This range is termed as **colour change interval of the indicator** (Table 2.5).

Table 2.5: Colour change of acid-base indicators.

Indicator	Transition pH range	Low pH color (Color in acidic solution)	High pH color (Color in basic solution)
Methyl yellow	2.9–4.0	Red	Yellow
Bromophenol blue	3.0–4.6	Yellow	Purple
Congo red	3.0–5.0	Blue-violet	Red
Methyl orange	3.1–4.4	Red	Yellow
Bromocresol green	3.8–5.4	Yellow	Blue-green
Methyl red	4.4–6.2	Red	Yellow
Bromocresol purple	5.2–6.8	Yellow	Purple
Bromocresol blue	6.0–7.6	Yellow	Blue
Phenol red	6.8–8.4	Yellow	Red
Neutral red	6.8–8.0	Red	Yellow
Thymol blue	8.0–9.6	Yellow	Blue
Naptholpthalein	7.3–8.7	Colorless	Greenish-blue
Phenolphthalein	8.3–10.1	Colorless	Pink
Thymolphthalein	9.3–10.5	Colorless	Blue

Theories of Acid Base Indicators

An acid-base indicator is an organic dye that signals the end point of the titration by a visual change in colour according to the hydrogen ion concentration (H^+). For most of the titrations it is possible to select indicators which exhibit a distinct colour change at a pH close to the equivalence pH. Three theories had been put forward to explain the indicator action in acid base titrations. These theories are discussed with the reference to commonly used indicators, namely litmus, methyl orange and phenolphthalein.

1. Litmus Theory

Litmus is a weak acid. It has a seriously complicated molecule which we will simplify to HLit. The "H" is the proton which can be given away to something else. The "Lit" is the rest of the weak acid molecule. There will be an equilibrium established when this acid dissolves in water. Taking the simplified version of this equilibrium:

$$HLit_{(aq)} \rightleftharpoons H_{(aq)} + Lit_{(aq)}$$

The un-ionized litmus is red, whereas the ion is blue. Now use Le-Chateliers principle to work out the change in colour if hydroxide ions or some more hydrogen ions are added to this equilibrium.

Adding Hydroxide Ions

Hydroxide ion reacts with the litmus and remove these hydrogen ions

$$HLit_{(aq)} \rightleftharpoons H^+_{(aq)} + Lit^-_{(aq)}$$

Litmus turns blue

The equilibrium position moves to replace the lost hydrogen ions

Adding Hydrogen Ions

Adding extra hydrogen ions

$$HLit_{(aq)} \rightleftharpoons H^+_{(aq)} + Lit^-_{(aq)}$$

Litmus turns red

The equilibrium position moves to replace the extra hydrogen ions

If the concentrations of HLit and Lit⁻ are equal: At some point during the movement of the position of equilibrium, the concentrations of the two colours will become equal. The colour observed will be a mixture of the two (neutral).

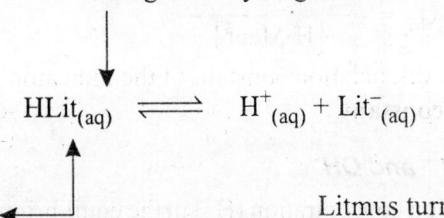

| Red | + | Blue | ⟶ | Netural |

The reason for the inverted commas around "neutral" is that there is no reason why the two concentrations should become equal at pH 7.

2. Ostwald theory: This theory is based on three postulates, viz;

(i) Acid-base indicator is a weak organic acid (HI_n) or a weak organic base, where the letter I_n^- is the complex organic group.

(ii) HI_n an unionized indicator, has a different colour from the I_n^- ions produced by the ionization of the indicator in the aqueous solution.

(iii) The degree of ionization of the indicator determines the visible colour of the indicator solution.

Illustration

Lets us take an example of **methyl orange** (pH range: 2.9–4.6) to explain the indicator action using Ostwald theory. The methyl orange is a weak acid and gives the following ionization equilibrium in solution as in the litmus case, but the colours are different.

$$\text{H-Meor} \rightleftharpoons \text{H}^+ + \text{Meor}^-$$

Applying law of mass action we get;

$$K_{In} = \frac{\left[H^+\right].\left[Meor^-\right]}{[\text{H-Meor}]}$$

Where K_{In} is a dissociation constant of the indicator and is called the **indicator constant**.

Addition of H⁺ and OH⁻

The hydrogen ion concentration $[H^+]$ in the equilibrium expression increases. To maintain K_{In} constant the equilibrium shifts to the left (according to the Le- Chateliers principle for the common ion effect). Thereby, the concentration of the $[In^-]$ is reduced and the concentration of [HIn] increases so that the colour of solution changes to red. On the other hand, upon the addition of the base to the solution, $[H^+]$ ions are removed as H_2O by reacting with OH⁻ ions of the base. This shifts the equilibrium to the right, resulting in increase of the $[In^-]$ ions that are yellow in colour (Fig. 2.9). In acid solution the unionized [HIn] molecules predominate and the solution is red (Fig. 2.10), while in basic solution the [In⁻] ions are in excess and the solution is yellow in colour as;

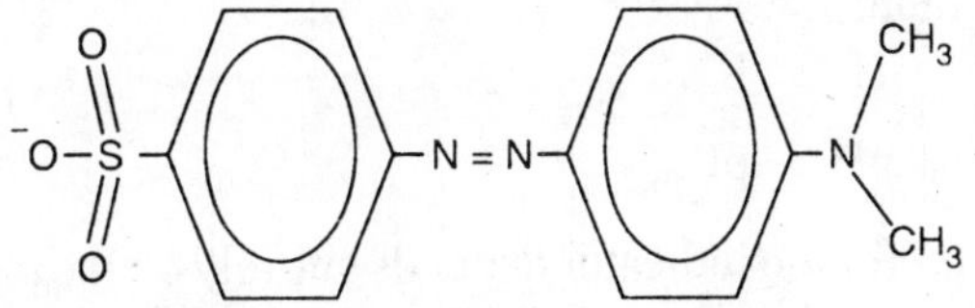

Fig. 2.9: *H-Meor (Yellow colour)*

When an acid is added, the hydrogen ion would be picked up by the negatively charged oxygen. In fact, the hydrogen ion attaches to one of the nitrogen's in the nitrogen-nitrogen double bond to give a structure which might be drawn like this:

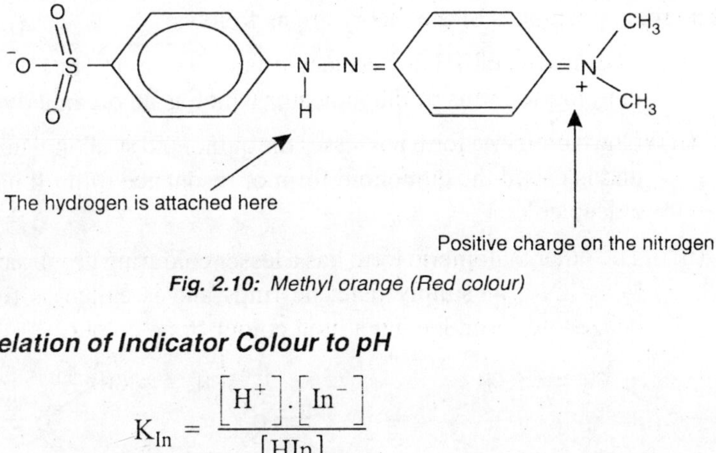

The hydrogen is attached here

Positive charge on the nitrogen

Fig. 2.10: *Methyl orange (Red colour)*

Relation of Indicator Colour to pH

$$K_{In} = \frac{\left[H^+\right].\left[In^-\right]}{[HIn]}$$

or $$[H^+] = \frac{\left[K_{In}\right].\left[In^-\right]}{[HIn]}$$

If the hydrogen ion concentration $[H^+]$ is large, the concentration of the [In⁻] ions is also higher and the colour is yellow but when the hydrogen ion concentration $[H^+]$ is less, the concentration of the [HIn] ions is more and the colour is red. At the equivalence point [In⁻] = [HIn] and the colour of the solution is **orange**. (Red + Yellow).The numerical valve of the K_{In} for the methyl orange is

3.7 and the pH of the orange solution is, therefore, about 4.0. If the last equation is re-arranged so that the hydrogen ion concentration is on the left-hand side, and then is converted to pH and pK_{ind}, then:

$$H^+ = K_{In}$$

$$pH = pK_{In}$$

The end point for the indicator depends entirely on the pK_{ind} value. For litmus, methyl orange and phenolphthalein the valve of pK_{In} is 6.5, 3.7 and 9.3, respectively (Table 2.6).

3. Quinonoid Theory

The Ostwald theory takes the quantitative aspect of the indicator action adequately but the cause for the colour change of an indicator in acid base solution is described by quinonoid theory of indicators. The main postulates of the theory are as follows;

(i)   The unionized $[H_2In]$ molecule and the anion $[In^{2-}]$ are tautomeric forms of the indicator which is an organic dye.

(ii) One tautomeric form possesses the quinonoid structural unit and is called the quinonoid form or resonance form. It has a deep colour.

(iii) The other tautomeric form has a lesser colouring group say, $[-N = N-]$ or simply benzene rings and is called as the benzenoid form, having a light colour or no colour.

Benzenoid form   Quinonoid form

(iv) The colour change of the indicator occurs when one tautomeric form is transformed into the other due to change in pH of the solution.

Illustration: Lets us take an example of **phenolphthalein** (pH range: 8.3–10.0) to explain the cause of colour of indicator. Phenolphthalein is weak acid and another commonly used indicator for acid/base titrations.

It is a diprotic acid, on losing first proton it gives a colourless form, but on loosing another proton, it forms an anion with conjugated system and a red-colour is produced.

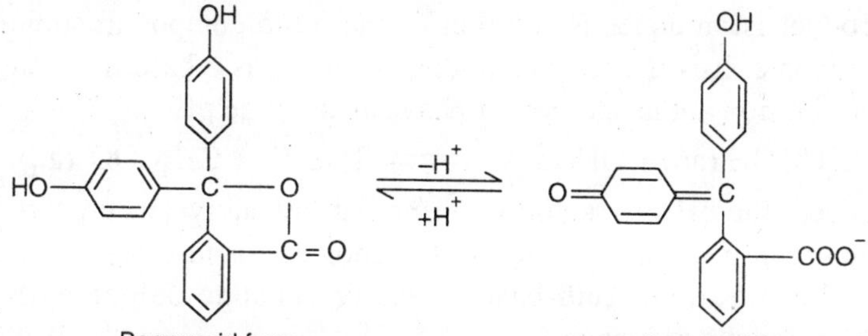

Benzenoid form
(colourless) (acidic medium)

Qunonoid form
(Pink) (alkaline medium)

Fig. 2.11: *Colour change in phenolphthalein.*

In this case, the weak acid is colourless and its ion is bright pink. Adding extra hydrogen ions shifts the position of equilibrium to the left, and turns the indicator colourless. Adding hydroxide ions removes the hydrogen ions from the equilibrium which tips to the right to replace them, turning the indicator pink (Fig. 2.11). The half-way stage happens at pH 9.3. Since a mixture of pink and colourless is simply a paler pink, this is difficult to detect with any accuracy. The exact values for the three indicators are looked as;

Table 2.6: *Indicators with their pK_{ind} and pH ranges.*

Indicator	pK_{ind}	pH range
Litmus	6.5	5–8
Methyl orange	3.7	3.1–4.4
Phenolphthalein	9.3	8.3–10.0
Phenol red	~7	6.8–8.4

2.13 Choice of Indicator in Acid Base Titration

Acid-base indicators take advantage of the rapid change in pH of the solution being titrated as the equivalence point is reached. When an acid and base have been mixed in equivalent amounts (according to the chemical equation for the reaction) they **neutralize** each other. However, this term is somewhat misleading because the pH of the solution depends on the salt formed, and may not be pH 7.

The choice of an indicator is determined by the pH of the solution at the equivalence point. At the equivalence point of a titration involving ethanoic acid and sodium hydroxide, the only product is an aqueous solution of the ionic compound sodium ethanoate. It is the ethanoate ions behaving as a base that cause the solution at the end-point to have an alkaline pH.

$$CH_3COOH \text{ (aq)} + OH^- \text{(aq)} \rightleftharpoons H_2O \text{ (l)} + CH_3COO^- \text{(aq)}$$

Indeed, the pH of a solution formed at the equivalence point is important because it influences the choice of acid-base indicator for the titration. Acid-base indicators change colour within characteristic pH ranges.

Choosing Indicators for Different Titrations

(1) Strong Acid and a Strong Base

The (Fig. 2.12) shows the pH curve for adding a strong acid to a strong base and superimposed on it are the pH ranges for methyl orange and phenolphthalein. In this curve neither of the indicator changes colour at the equivalence point. However, the graph is so

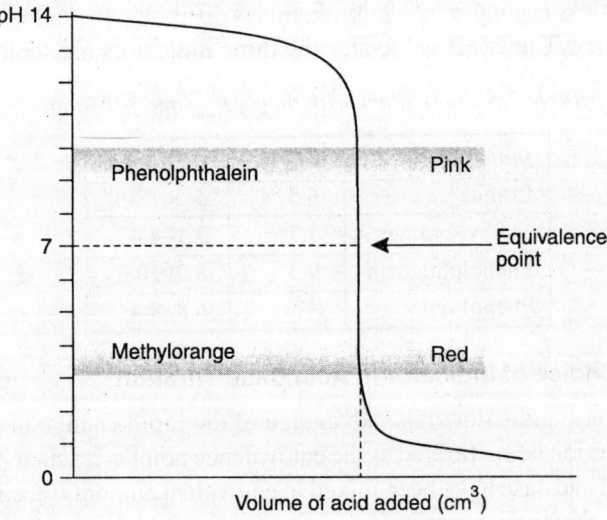

Fig. 2.12: *pH curve for titrating a strong acid with a strong base.*

steep at that point that there will be virtually no difference in the volume of acid added whichever indicator is choosen. However, it would make sense to titrate to the best possible colour with each indicator. If Phenolphthalein is used, titration is carried out until it just becomes colourless (at pH 8.3) because that is as close as the equivalence point. On the other hand, using methyl orange, titration is carried out until there is the very first trace of orange in the solution. If the solution becomes red, it is more close to equivalence point.

(2) Strong Acid and a Weak Base

The (Fig. 2.13) showing a curve in which phenolphthalein would be completely useless. However, methyl orange starts to change from yellow towards orange very close to the equivalence point. An indicator is choosen which changes colour on the steep bit of the curve.

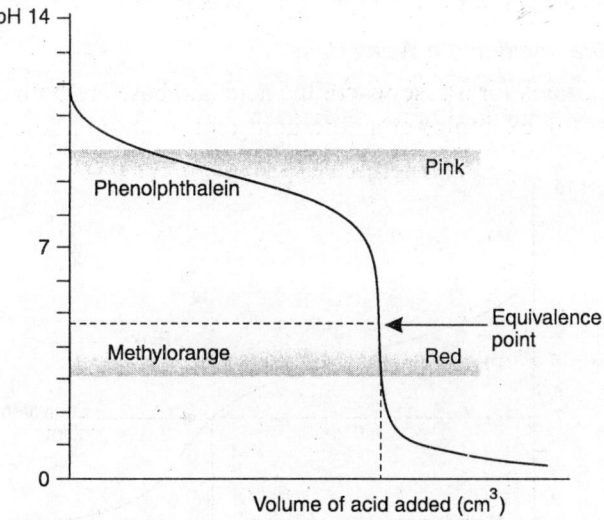

Fig. 2.13: *pH curve for titrating a strong acid with a weak base.*

(3) Weak Acid and a Strong Base

In titrating weak acid with a strong base, methyl orange is useless. However, the phenolphthalein changes colour exactly when titration is carried out (Fig. 2.14).

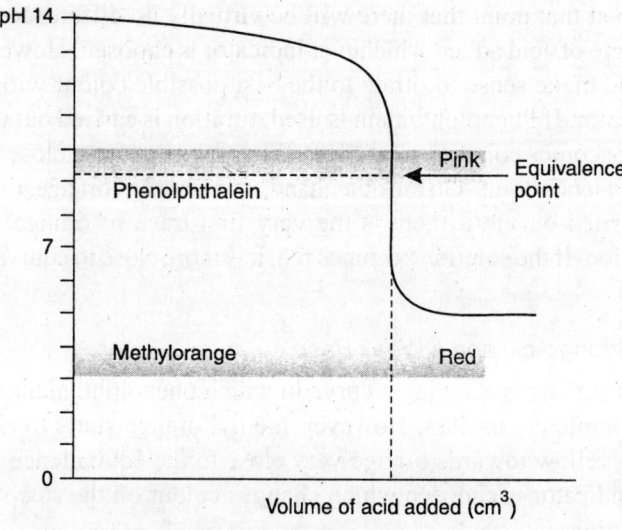

Fig. 2.14: pH curve for titrating a weak acid with a strong base.

(4) Weak Acid and a Weak Base

The curve is for a case where the acid and base are both equally weak, for example, ethanoic acid and ammonia solution. If

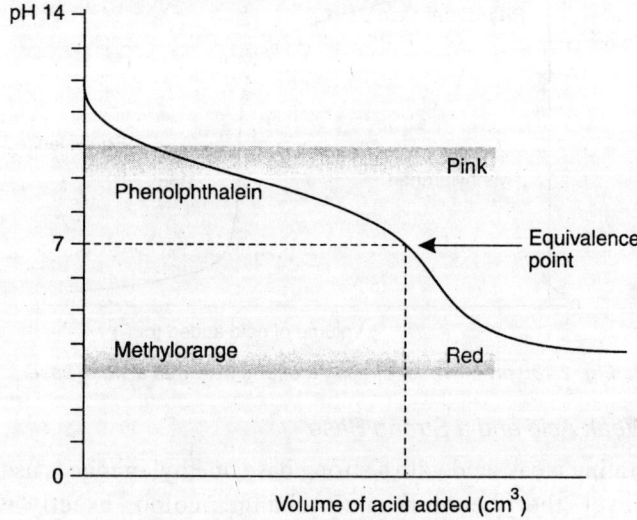

Fig. 2.15: pH curve for titrating a weak acid with a weak base.

phenolphthalein or methyl orange is used, both will give a valid titration result, but the value with phenolphthalein will be exactly half the methyl orange (Fig. 2.15).

It may be possible to find an indicator which starts to change color at the equivalence point, but because the pH of the equivalence point will be different from case to case, it cannot be generalized.

On the whole titration a weak acid and a weak base should not be carried out in the presence of an indicator, e.g., sodium carbonate solution and dilute hydrochloric acid.

Phenolphthalein will finish changing well before the equivalence point, and methyl orange falls off the graph altogether. It so happens that the phenolphthalein has finished its colour change at exactly the pH of the equivalence point of the first half of the reaction in which sodium hydrogen carbonate is produced (Fig. 2.16).

$$Na_2CO_{3(aq)} + HCl_{(aq)} \longrightarrow NaCl_{(aq)} + NaHCO_{3(aq)}$$

The methyl orange changes colour at exactly the pH of the equivalence point of the second stage of the reaction.

$$NaHCO_{3(aq)} + HCl_{(aq)} \longrightarrow NaCl_{(aq)} + CO_{2(g)} + H_2O_{(l)}$$

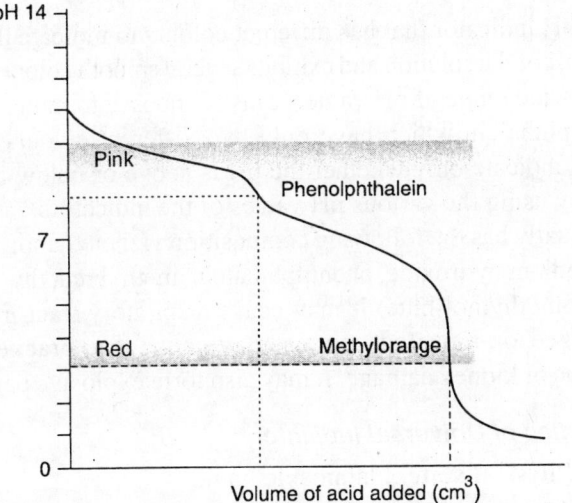

Fig. 2.16: *pH curve for weak base and weak acid in the presence of methyl orange and phenolphthalein*

Table 2.7: *Choice of acid-base indicators*

Titration	Indicator	pH range of colour change	Titrant
Strong acid and Strong base	Phenolphthalein	5–9	Alkali
	Methyl orange		Acid
Strong acid and Weak base	Methyl orange	4	Acid
Weak acid and Strong base	Phenolphthalein	8	Alkali
Weak acid and Weak base	Phenol red	~7	Alkali

2.14 Universal Indicator

It is a pH indicator that has different colours to indicate the range of the pH of the solution and exhibits several smooth colour changes over a wide range of pH values. This is opposed to indicators like phenolphthalein which have only two different colours and are able to indicate only whether the pH is above or below a certain point by using the various pH values of the indicators.

It usually has the following composition viz; methanol, propan-1-ol, sodium hydroxide, phenolphthalein, methyl red, thymol blue and bromothymol blue. It may cause respiratory tract irritation. Prolonged or repeated contact may cause dry, cracked skin, irritation or kidney damage. It may also form explosive peroxides.

Properties of Universal Indicator

1. **Physical state**: Flammable liquid.
2. **Appearance**: Light green in water solvent; dark green alone.
3. **Odour**: Alcohol-like

4. **pH value**: Approximately 7
5. **Vapour pressure**: 25 mmHg (3.3 kPa)
6. **Vapour density**: 1.3 kg/m³
7. **Molecular formula**: Mixture
8. **Boiling point**: 80 °C
9. **Solubility**: Soluble in water.
10. **Specific gravity/density**: 0.93 g/cm³

Preparation of Universal Indicator

Dissolve 0.1 g of phenolphthalein + 0.2 g of methyl red + 0.3 g of methyl yellow + 0.4 g of bromothymol blue + 0.5 g of thymol blue in 500 ml of absolute methanol or propan-1-ol and add NaOH solution until the **color** of solution is dark green.

2.15 Polyprotic Systems

Polyprotic systems are compounds that can donate or accept more than one proton.

Polyprotic Acids

Polyprotic acids are able to donate more than one proton per acid molecule, in contrast to monoprotic acids that only donate one proton per molecule.

Specific types of polyprotic acids have more specific names, such as **diprotic acid** (two potential protons to donate) and **triprotic acid** (three potential protons to donate).

A monoprotic acid can undergo dissociation (sometimes called ionization) as follows and simply has one acid dissociation constant as shown below:

$$HA\ (aq) + H_2O\ (l) \rightleftharpoons H_3O^+(aq) + A^-(aq)\ K_a$$

A diprotic acid (here symbolized by H_2A) can undergo one or two dissociations depending on the pH. Each dissociation has its own dissociation constant, K_{a1} and K_{a2}.

$$H_2A\ (aq) + H_2O\ (l) \rightleftharpoons H_3O^+(aq) + HA^-(aq)\ K_{a1}$$

$$HA^-(aq) + H_2O\ (l) \rightleftharpoons H_3O^+(aq) + A^{2-}(aq)\ K_{a2}$$

The first dissociation constant is typically greater than the second, i.e., $K_{a1} > K_{a2}$. For example, sulfuric acid (H_2SO_4) can donate one proton to form the bisulfate anion (HSO_4^-), for which K_{a1} is very large; then it can donate a second proton to form the sulfate anion (SO_4^{2-}), wherein the K_{a2} is intermediate strength.

The large K_{a1} for the first dissociation makes sulfuric acid a strong acid. In a similar manner, the weak unstable carbonic acid (H_2CO_3) can lose one proton to form bicarbonate anion (HCO_3^-) and lose a second to form carbonate anion (CO_3^{2-}). Both K_a values are small, but $K_{a1} > K_{a2}$.

A triprotic acid (H_3A) can undergo one, two, or three dissociations and has three dissociation constants, where $K_{a1} > K_{a2} > K_{a3}$.

$$H_3A\ (aq) + H_2O\ (l) \rightleftharpoons H_3O^+\ (aq) + H_2A^-\ (aq)\ K_{a1}$$

$$H_2A^-\ (aq) + H_2O\ (l) \rightleftharpoons H_3O^+\ (aq) + HA^{2-}\ (aq)\ K_{a2}$$

$$HA^{2-}\ (aq) + H_2O\ (l) \rightleftharpoons H_3O^+\ (aq) + A^{3-}\ (aq)\ K_{a3}$$

In contrast to a simple monoprotic acid like acetic acid with single equilibrium between the acid and conjugate base, a polyprotic acid contains more than one acidic hydrogen. For a polyprotic acid, n acidic hydrogen's will exist in solution in equilibrium with n conjugate base forms (for a total of $n + 1$ species). For example, when phosphoric acid ($n = 3$, a triprotic acid) is dissolved in solution, the following equilibriums are established among the four species H_3PO_4 (phosphoric acid itself), $H_2PO_4^{-1}$ (dihydrogen phosphate anion), HPO_4^{2-} (hydrogen phosphate anion), and PO_4^{-3} (Phosphate ion) (Fig. 2.17).

$$H_3PO_a + H_2O \rightleftharpoons H_2PO_a^- + H_3O^+ \qquad K_{a1} = \frac{[H_2PO_4^-][H_3O^+]}{[H_3PO_4]} = 7.5 \times 10^{-3}$$

$$H_2PO_4^- + H_2O \rightleftharpoons HPO_4^{-2} + H_3O^+ \qquad K_{a2} = \frac{[HPO_4^{-2}][H_3O^+]}{[H_3PO_4^-]} = 6.23 \times 10^{-8}$$

$$HPO_4^{-2} + H_2O \rightleftharpoons PO_4^{-3} + H_3O^+ \qquad K_{a3} = \frac{[PO_4^{3-}][H_3O^+]}{[HPO_4^{-2}]} = 2.2 \times 10^{-13}$$

Fig. 2.17: Dissociation of phosphoric acid- A triprotic acid.

Another important example of a triprotic acid is citric acid, which can successively lose three protons to finally form the citrate ion. Even though the positions of the protons on the original molecule may be equivalent, the successive K_a values will differ since it is energetically less favorable to lose a proton if the conjugate base is more negatively charged.

2.16 Neutralization or Acid-Base Titration Curves

Acid-base titrations are often recorded on titration curves which is drawn by plotting data obtained during a titration in which, titrant volume is plotted on the x-axis (ordinate) and pH or pOH on the y-axis (absicae). The independent variable is the volume of the titrant, while the dependent variable is the pH or pOH of the solution (which changes depending on the composition of the two solutions). Important parts of titration curve are:

1. **The buffering region**: The resulting lag that precedes the equivalence point is called the buffering region. In this region it takes a large amount of titrant to produce a small change in pH or pOH of the receiving solution.

2. **The equivalence point:** It is a significant point on the graph at which, all of the starting solution, usually an acid has been neutralized by the titrant, usually a base. It can be calculated precisely by finding the second derivative of the titration curve

3. **The point of inflection**: It is a point on titration curve where the graph changes its concavity.

In acid base titration curve, the valve of pH or pOH rises slowly at the start of the titration, but rapidly increases as the equivalence point is reached (from 3.3–10.7) and increases slowly after the elapse of equivalence point. In other words rate of change of pH of the solution at equivalence point is very fast.

The Titration Curve of a Strong Acid Against a Strong Base

The titration of a strong acid (0.1M HCl) with a strong base (0.1M NaOH) produces the titration curve given in fig. 2.19.

$$HCl = [H^+]$$
$$[0.1 \text{ m}] = [0.1 \text{ m}]$$
$$= 10^{-1} \text{ ions/litre}$$
$$\therefore \quad pH = -\log [H^+]$$
$$= -\log [10^{-1}]$$

or $\qquad pH = 1$

Therefore the curve will start from pH = 1 and the equivalence point for a strong acid-strong base titration curve is exactly 7 because the salt produced does not undergo any hydrolysis reactions.

The outline of the titration curve for acid base titration is given as in fig.2.18 below;

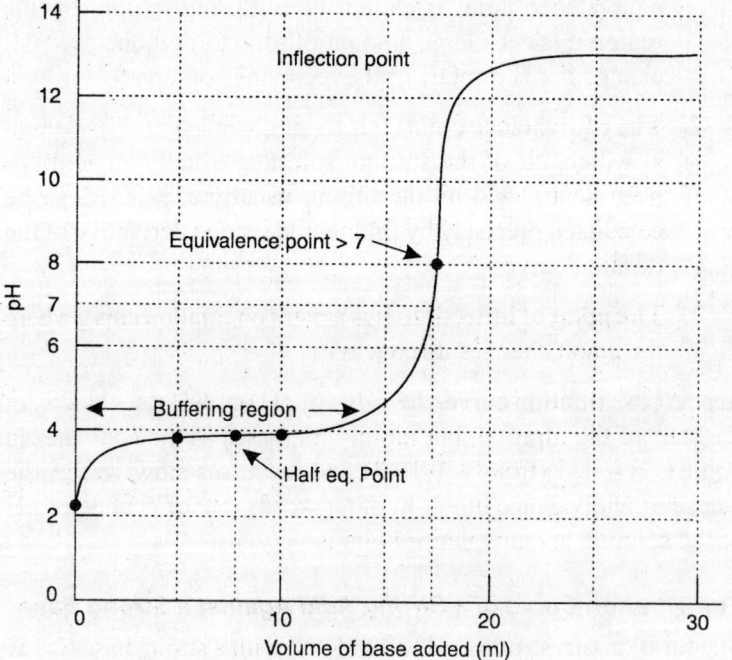

Fig. 2.18: *Titration curve of acid/base titration.*

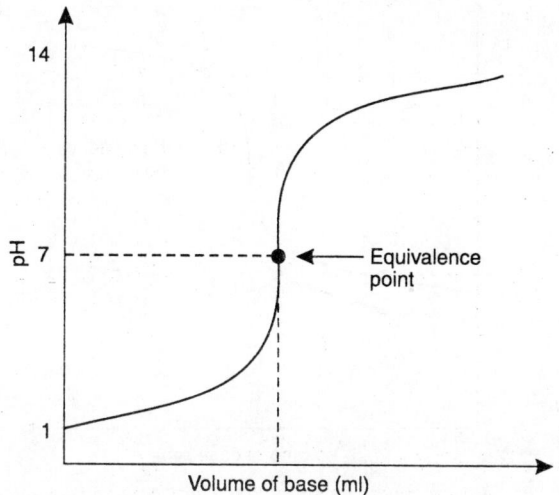

Fig. 2.19: *Titration curve of a strong base titrating with a strong acid.*

Titration Curve of a Strong Base Titrating Against Weak Acid

If a strong base is used to titrate against weak acid, the pH at the equivalence point will not be 7. There is a lag in reaching the equivalence point, as some of the weak acid is converted to its conjugate base. The pair of a weak acid and its conjugate base is known as a buffer.

In (Fig. 2.20) the resultant lag that precedes the equivalence point is called the **buffering region**. In the buffering region, it takes a large amount of titrant to produce a small change in the pH of the receiving solution. Due to basic nature of the conjugate base, the pH will be greater than 7 at the equivalence point.

The pH is calculated by using the Henderson-Hasselbalch equation, and inputting the pK_b and concentration of the conjugate base of the weak acid. The titration of a base with an acid produces a flipped-over version of the titration curve of an acid with a base.

2.17 Mixed Indicators

Mixed indicators are actually mixtures of suitable acid-base indicators used in acid base titrations. These are used in those

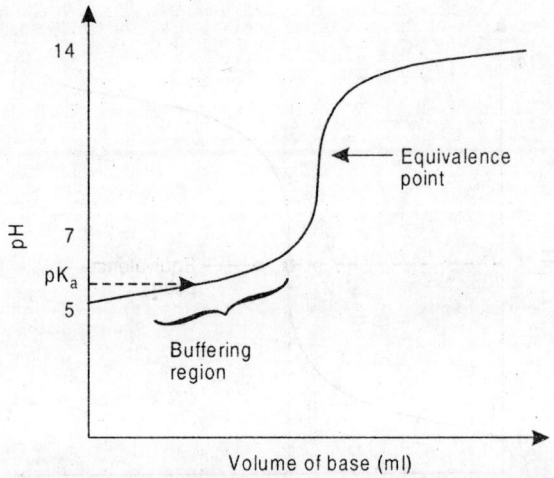

Fig. 2.20: *Titration curve of a strong base titrating against weak acid*

cases, where a sharp colour change is required over a narrow and selected range of pH. While preparing mixed indicators, it must be kept in mind that

1. The pK_{in} values of the selected acid-base indicators are close together and

2. The over lapping colours are complementary at an intermediate pH valves.

For example bromocresol green (pk_{in}–4.9) and methyl red (pk_{in}–5.0) give a red colour in acid and green color in alkaline media with a sharp transition through grey at pH=5.1 as the two colors of indicators are complementary.

Some Important Examples

1. Neutral red and methylene blue: This mixture has equal parts of 1% solution of neutral red in ethanol and 1% of methylene blue in ethanol. The equivalence point is obtained at pH = 7.

2. Phenolphthalein and 1-naphtholphthalein: A mixture of 1% pure solution of the phenolphthalein in ethanol and 1% solution of 1 naptholpthalein in ethanol in a ratio 3:1 serves as good mixed indicator. The equivalence point is obtained at pH = 8.9 as it passes from pale rose to violet. This is suitable for the titration of phosphoric acid (H_3PO_4) to the dynamic stage.

3. Thymol blue and cresol red: A mixture of 1% aqueous solution of sodium salt of thymol blue and 1% of aqueous solution of sodium salt of cresol red in ratio of 3:1. The equivalence point is obtained at pH = 8.3 as it passes from yellow to violet. It is used for the titration of carbonate to the HCO_3^- stage.

4. Xylene cyanol and methyl orange: It is a mixture of 1.4 g of xylene cyanol and 1 g of methyl orange in 500 ml of 50% ethanol and gives colour change from alkaline medium to acid medium as green → gray → purple red. The equivalence point is obtained at pH = 3.8. This is also called 'screened' methyl orange.

2.18 Important Assays in Acid Base Titration

1. Acidimetry Titration

(A) Direct titration

(i) Assay of sodium bicarbonate:

I.P limit: It contains not less than 99% and not more the equivalent of 100.5% $NaHCO_3$ calculated with reference to the dried substance.

Procedure: Accurately weigh about 1 g of $NaHCO_3$ and dissolve in 20 ml of distilled water. Titrate the solution with 0.5 N sulphuric acid using methyl orange as an indicator. The end point is reached when yellow colour is changed into pink colour.

$$2\,NaHCO_3 + H_2SO_4 \longrightarrow Na_2SO_4 + 2\,H_2O + 2\,CO_2$$

In the assay of $NaHCO_3$, phenolphthalein is not used as indicator because it causes early detection of end point due to the production of carbonic acid during the reaction.

Factor: 1m l. of 0.5 NH_2SO_4 is equivalent to 0.042 g of $NaHCO_3$.

(ii) Assay of Sodium Carbonate

I.P limit: It contains not less than 99% and not more than the equivalent of 105% of $Na_2CO_3\,10\,H_2O$.

Theory: Sodium carbonate is alkaline in nature. It is assayed by titrating with a standard acid using bromophenol blue as an indicator. At the end point, acidic pH is obtained due to formation of carbonic acid from carbon dioxide.

$$Na_2CO_3 + H_2SO_4 \longrightarrow Na_2SO_4 + H_2O + CO_2$$

Procedure: Weigh accurately sodium carbonate (2 g), dissolve in water (20 ml) and titrate with 0.5 N sulphuric acid by using bromophenol as an indicator. The end point is reached when the colour of solution turns yellow.

Factor: Each ml of 0.5 N H_2SO_4 is equivalent to 0.0715 g of Na_2CO_3.

(B) Residual Titration

(i) Assay of Strong Ammonia Solution

I.P limit: It contains not less than 24.5% w/w and not more than 25.5% w/w of NH_3.

Theory: The ammonia solution being volatile in nature. It is assayed by residual or back titration. Ammonia solution is treated with an accurately measured standard acid and the acid is back titrated with a standard alkali by using methyl red as an indicator.

$$2\,NH_3 + H_2SO_4 \longrightarrow (NH_4)_2\,SO_4$$

Ammonia   Diammonium sulphate

Procedure: Weigh accurately ammonia solution (3 g) in a flask containing 1 N sulphuric acid (50 ml) and titrate the excess of acid with 1 N sodium hydroxide solution by using methyl red as an indicator. The end point is reached when yellow colour is changed to red colour.

Factor: Each ml of 1N H_2SO_4 is equivalent to 0.01703 g of NH_3.

(ii) Assay of Zinc Oxide

I.P limit: It contains not less than 99% and not more than the equivalent of 100.5% of ZnO, calculated with reference to the ignited substance.

Procedure: Accurately weigh 1.5 g of zinc oxide and 2.5 g of ammonium chloride. Mix and dissolve the solution in 1 N sulphuric acid solution (50 ml) with the aid of gentle heating. Titrate the required solution with 1N sodium hydroxide using bromophenol as an indicator. The end point is reached when colour of the solution turns yellow.

$$ZnO + H_2SO_4 \longrightarrow ZnSO_4 + H_2O.$$

Factor: Each ml of 1N H_2SO_4 is equivalent to 0.04068 g of ZnO.

2. Alkalimetry Titration

(A) Direct Titration

(i) Estimation of Boric Acid

IP Limit: It contains not less than 99% and not more than 100.5% of boric acid (H_3BO_3) with reference to dried substances.

Theory: Boric acid is a weak acid hence can't be titrated directly with dissolving in a solution of glycerin in water. The boric acid reacts with glycerin to form glyceryl boric acid which is strong monobasic acid. The glycerol is slightly acidic in nature, therefore, it is neutralized with dilute alkali using phenolphthalein indicator.

$$H_3BO_3 = NaOH = 1000 \text{ ml NaOH}$$
$$61.84 \text{ g } H_3BO_3 = 1000 \text{ ml NaOH}$$
$$0.0618 = 1 \text{ ml M NaOH}$$

$\therefore$ Each 1 ml of 1 M NaOH 0.0618 g of H_3BO_3.

Procedure: Weight accurately 0.25 g of H_3BO_3 and dissolve it in a mixture of 6.5 ml distilled H_2O and 12.5 ml of glycerin. Titrate the required solution with 0.1N NaOH using phenolphthalein as Indicator. The pink colour is obtained at end point.

Factor: Each 1 ml of or 1 M NaOH is equivalent to 0.0618 g of H_3BO_3

Preparation of 0.1N NaOH

$$\text{Equivalent wt} = \frac{NaOH}{Basicity} = \frac{40}{1} = 40 \text{ g}$$

Weigh accurately 40 g of NaOH and dissolve it in 1000 ml distilled water = 1 N

For 0.1 N $\rightarrow$ Weigh accurately 4 g of NaOH solution and dissolve it 250 ml of distilled water. Make up the volume up to 1000 ml in a volumetric flask.

Standardization: With HCl: Pipette 20 ml of 0.1 N NaOH solution into a conical flask, add 2 drops of phenolphthalein and titrate with N/10 HCl, the solution changes to colourless at the end point. Note burette reading for calculating the normality of NaOH solution.

$$N_{NaOH} \times V_{NaOH} = N_{HCl} \times V_{HCl}$$

(ii) Assay of Ammonium Chloride

I.P limit: It contains not less than 99.5% of NH_4Cl, calculated with reference to the dried substance.

Procedure: Weigh accurately ammonium chloride (about 0.1g), dissolve in water (20 ml) and add formaldehyde solution (5 ml) previously neutralized to phenolphthalein indicator. Titrate the solution with 0.1 N sodium hydroxide solution (NaOH) using phenolphthalein as an indicator. The end point is reached when pink coloured solution is obtained.

Factor: Each 1 ml of 0.1 N NaOH is equivalent to 0.005349 g of NH_4Cl.

(B) Residual Titration

In such titrations the acid is treated with excess of accurately measured base which is then back titrated with a standard acid.

(i) Assay of Aspirin

I.P limit: It contains not less than 99.5% and not more than the equivalent of 100.5% of aspirin.

Procedure: Weigh accurately aspirin (1.5 g) and add 0.5 N sodium hydroxide (50 ml). Boil the solution for 10 minutes. Cool it and titrate the excess of alkali with 0.5 N sulphuric acid solution using phenol red as an indicator. Perform a blank titration in the same way. The liberated acid reacts with sodium hydroxide to form sodium salt. At the end point, a slight excess of the base reacts with the indicator to produce colour change.

Factor: Each 1 ml of 0.5 N NaOH is equivalent to 0.04504 g of $C_9 H_8 O_4$.

EXERCISES

1. Discuss briefly about Lewis concept of acids and bases.
2. State law of mass action, derive the equation and write its applications.
3. What is pH, derive the equation of pH for pure water and write its applications?
4. Write a note on relative strength of acids and bases.
5. What are buffer solutions? How do they regulate pH change?
6. Derive the Henderson's Hasselbalch equation for weak acid and its salt.
7. Write a note on hydrolysis of salt. Derive the equation for hydrolysis constant.
8. Write a note on common ion effect. What is its importance?
9. What is polyprotic system? Derive equation for dissociation of polyprotic system.
10. Describe the theory of acid/base indicators in details.
11. Give the role of solvents in acid/base titrations.
12. What is neutralization curve? Draw the titration curve between strong acid and strong base.
13. What are acid base indicators? Give the parameters required for choosing acid base indicator.
14. What are mixed indicators? Mention some examples and assays for which they are required.
15. Discuss the effect of acids, temperature and solvents upon the solubility of precipitate.
16. 0.22g of $KHCO_3$ was titrated against 0.1N HCl (21 ml of acid was used). Calculate percentage purity of sample (Eq.wt of $KHCO_3$ = 100.5g).
17. Calculate the pH for 0.1 M HCl.
18. Discuss the estimation of boric acid. Calculate pH for 2g of NaOH.
19. What is titration curve? Discuss titration curve for the neutralization of:
    (i) Strong acid and strong base.
    (ii) Weak acid and weak base.

20. Explain the colour of phenolphthalein and methyl orange in different solution using acid/base indicator theory.

21. Explain why do the solution of weak acid and its salt behave as a buffer, but a solution of strong acid and its salt does not.

22. Differentiate between direct and indirect acid/base titration. Explain with examples.

23. Describe salt hydrolysis in detail.

24. What do you mean by following expression: pH + pOH = 14. The pH of the solution is 8. Calculate its hydrogen ion and hydroxyl ion concentration.

25. Explain the titration curve of the polyprotic systems in detail.

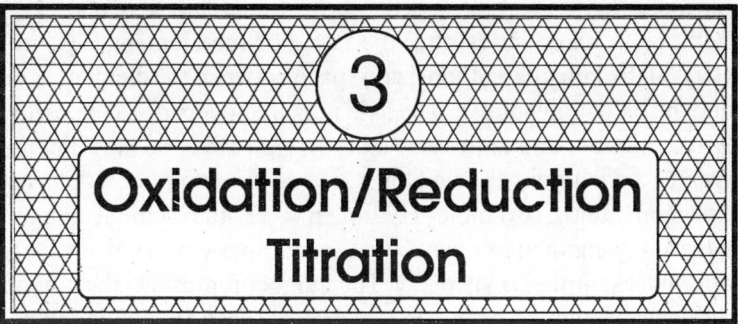

3

Oxidation/Reduction Titration

A quantitative method of analysis in which volume of a sample solution is determined by titrating it against standard oxidising or reducing agent using redox indicators is called as oxidation reduction titration. The oxidation reduction titration involves redox reactions, i.e., the process in which oxidation and reduction occurs simultaneously. It is also defined as a volumetric analysis that relies on a net change in the oxidation number of one or more species.

3.1 Terms Involved in Oxidation Reduction Titration

1. Oxidation: A process which involves the loss of one or more electrons by an atom (de-electronation), molecules or ions.

2. Reduction: A process which involves the gain of one or more electron by an atom (electronation), molecules or ions.

$$Fe^{2+} \longrightarrow Fe^{3+} + e^-$$
(Ferrous ion)   (Ferric)   (Loss of electron)

$$Ce^{3+} \longrightarrow Ce^{4+} + e^- \qquad \text{(Oxidation)}$$

$$Fe^{3+} + e^- \longrightarrow Fe^{2+}$$
(Ferric ion)   (Gain of   (Ferrous ion)
                  electron)

$$Ce^{4+} + e^- \longrightarrow Ce^{3+} \qquad \text{(Reduction)}$$

3. Oxidation number: It is the charge of an element in a molecule or complex after oxidation or reduction. The oxidation number is placed either as a right superscript to the element symbol, e.g., Fe^{III}, or in parentheses after the name of the element, e.g., iron (III): in the latter case, there is no space between the element name and the oxidation number. The oxidation number can also be written with a number and either a +ve or -ve sign after it. If the element creates a positively charged ion, the oxidation number will have a +ve sign after it, (example- Hydrogen 1^{+}). If the element creates a negatively charged ion, the oxidation number will have a -ve sign after it, (example-Oxygen 2^{-}). The number represents the number of electrons gained or lost in a chemical reaction. Oxidation and reduction properly refer to a change in **oxidation number**, the actual transfer of electrons may never occur. Thus, oxidation is better defined as an **increase** in oxidation number, and reduction as a **decrease** in oxidation number. In practice, the transfer of electrons will always cause a change in oxidation number, but there are many reactions which are classed as redox even though no electron transfer occurs.

4. Oxidation state: In chemistry, the **oxidation state** is an indicator of the degree of oxidation of an atom in a chemical compound. The formal oxidation state is the hypothetical charge that an atom would have if all bonds to atoms of different elements were 100% ionic. Oxidation states are represented by positive, negative, or zero. Thus, H^{+} would have an oxidation state of 1+. The increase in oxidation state of an atom is known as an **oxidation** while as a decrease in oxidation state is known as a **reduction**. Such reactions involve the transfer of electrons, a net gain in electrons being a reduction and a net loss of electrons being an oxidation.

5. A reducing agent: An agent that losses electrons and is oxidised.

6. An oxidising agent: An agent that gains electrons and is reduced.

$$Fe^{2+} \longrightarrow Fe^{3+} + e^{-}$$

(Reducing agent)　　(Oxidising agent)

Now the electron loosed by reducing agent is gained by the oxidising agent. Therefore, there is an increase in the electro-negative portion of the molecule. Hence, atoms converted into a higher state of oxidation.

$$Fe^{2+} \longrightarrow Fe^{3+} + e^- \text{ (electronegative}$$
$$\downarrow \qquad \text{portion of molecule)}$$

(Higher state of oxidation)

7. Oxidation reduction reaction: A combination of oxidising and reducing agents results in oxidation-reduction reaction which forms the basis for the quantitative measurement of one of the reactants. It is also called as **redox reaction** as 'redox' is the abbreviated form of reduction-oxidation system. A typical example of redox reaction in which a ferric salt is reduced by a titanous salt is given as;

$$TiCl_3 + FeCl_3 \longrightarrow TiCl_4 + FeCl_2$$

(Titanous chloride)

The equation can be written is an ionic form as:

$$Ti^{3+} + Fe^{3+} \longrightarrow Ti^{4+} + Fe^{2+}$$

(Oxidised)   (Reduced)

Hence, one agent or reactant can be easily estimated by titrating with other agent. This may be separated into two-half equation, one of which represents oxidation and other reduction as:

$$Ti^{3+} \rightleftharpoons Ti^{4+} + e^-$$

$$Fe^{3+} + e^- \rightleftharpoons Fe^{2+}$$

Hence, $KMnO_4$ (an oxidising agent) is used for the estimation of $FeSO_4$ (a reducing agent) and $Na_2S_2O_3$ (a reducing agent) is used for the estimation of I_2 (an oxidising agent).

8. Redox Indicator: A redox indicator is an organic dye which signals the completion of redox reaction or titration by the visual color change at a specific electrode potential. E.g., Starch, $KMnO_4$, Potassium ferricyanide etc.

3.2 Nernst Equation

The equation gives the relationship between electrode potential (E) of any given redox system, concentration of oxidised/reduced forms and shows the dependence of electrode potential on concentration. Consider a reversible redox system:

Oxidant + ne $\rightleftharpoons$ Reductant

When an inert (or unattackable) electrode is introduced, the established electrode potential is given by:

$$E_T = E° + \frac{RT}{nF} \ln \frac{[Ox]}{Red} \qquad ...(i)$$

$E°$ = Standard electrode (or reduction) potential
E_T = Potential observed at absolute temperature (T)
R = Gas constant = 8.314 Joules/deg/mol^{-1}
F = Faraday's constant = 96500 coulombs
T = Absolute temperature = 298°K (25°C) and
n = number of electrons gained by an oxidant in being converted to the reducing agent.

Converting equation (i) to common logarithm and expressing in terms of concentration we get;

$$E_{25} = E° + \frac{0.0591}{n} \log \frac{[Ox]}{Red} \qquad ...(ii)$$

i.e., the electrode potential of a system can be calculated from the knowledge of $E°$ and percentage of oxidised and reduced forms present. The equation (ii) is called **Nernst equation** and if the term $\log \dfrac{[Ox]}{Red}$ is unity, then E is equal to $E°$ and is called **standard electrode (or reduction) potential of an electrode.** The concentration is approximately unity for a 1 M solution.

E.g., For Permanganate / Manganese [MnO_4^- / Mn^{+2}] system =

$$E_{25} = 1.52 + \frac{0.0591}{5} \log \frac{\left[MnO_4^-\right]}{\left[Mn^{+2}\right]}$$

Hence, **strength** of oxidising and reducing agent depends on standard electrode potential ($E°$) and capacity of that agent to oxidize and reduce. Few examples of redox systems with their $E°$ valve are depicted in (Fig. 3.1) as;

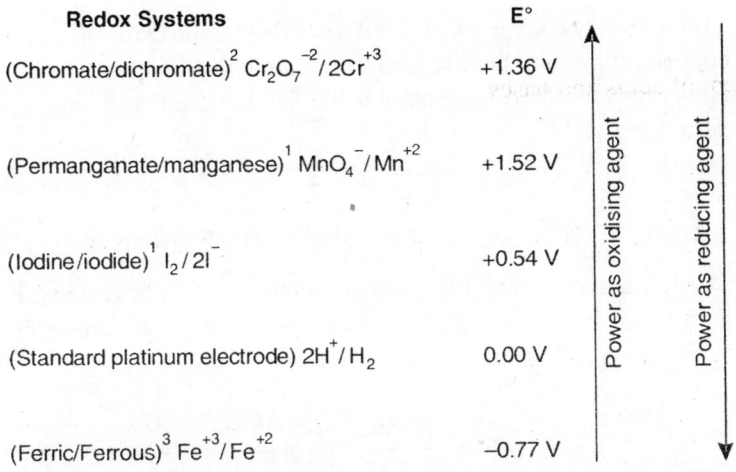

Fig. 3.1: *Redox systems and their standard electrode potential (E°).*

The E^o is a quantitative measure of the tendency of element to lose electron, and thus measures the strength of element as reducing agent in aqueous solution. The greater the negative (- ve) valve of potential of an element, the more strongly it functions as reducing agent.

3.3 Equilibrium Constant of Redox Systems

Using the Nernst equation the valve of equilibrium constant (K) for the redox reaction can be calculated, and thereby it may be determined whether such reaction can be of use in titrimetric procedure. Consider the following, a complex redox duplex reaction:

$$10\ FeSO_4 + 2KMnO_4 + 8H_2SO_4 \longrightarrow 5Fe_2(SO_4)_3 + 2MnSO_4$$
$$+ K_2SO_4 + 4H_2O$$

Ionic form: $5\ Fe^{2+} + MnO_4^- + 8H^+ \rightleftharpoons 5Fe^{3+} + Mn^{2+} + 4H_2O$

Applying law of mass action: ...(i)

$$K = \frac{\left[Mn^{2+}\right]\left[Fe^{3+}\right]^5}{\left[MnO_4^-\right]\left[H^+\right]^8\left[Fe^{2+}\right]^5}$$

Since the reaction is carried in dilute solution, the H_2O concentration may be assumed to remain constant, the term H_2O is therefore omitted for equation (i). The two half reactions may be written as;

$$5\ Fe^{2+} \rightleftharpoons 5\ Fe^{3+} + e^- \quad \text{[Oxidation half]}$$

$$KMnO_4^- + 8H^+ + 5e^- \rightleftharpoons Mn^{2+} + 4H_2O \quad \text{[Reduction half]}$$

In such a redox reaction permanganate ion is converted into manganese ion by gaining 5 electrons. Therefore, applying Nernst equation on reduction half as;

$$E = E_0 + \frac{0.0591}{5} \log \frac{\left[MnO_4^-\right]\left[H^+\right]^8}{\left[Mn^{2+}\right]}$$

$$E = 1.52 + \frac{0.0591}{5} \log \frac{\left[MnO_4^-\right]\left[H^+\right]^8}{\left[Mn^{2+}\right]}$$

Nernst equation on oxidation half as;

$$E = E_0 + \frac{0.0591}{5} \log \frac{\left[Fe^{3+}\right]^5}{\left[Fe^{2+}\right]^5}$$

$$E = 0.77 + \frac{0.0591}{5} \log \frac{\left[Fe^{3+}\right]^5}{\left[Fe^{2+}\right]^5}$$

When equilibrium is reached, the net e.m.f of the cell will be zero, or, the potential of the two electrodes will be equal.

$$1.52 + \frac{0.0591}{5} \log \frac{\left[MnO_4^-\right]\left[H^+\right]^8}{\left[Mn^{2+}\right]} = 0.77 + \frac{0.0591}{5}$$

$$\log \frac{\left[Fe^{3+}\right]^5}{\left[Fe^{2+}\right]^5}$$

$$\log \frac{\left[Mn^{2+} \right]\left[Fe^{3+} \right]^5}{\left[MnO_4^- \right]\left[H^+ \right]^8 \left[Fe^{2+} \right]^5} = \frac{5\left[1.52 - 0.77 \right]}{0.0591}$$

$$\log \frac{\left[Mn^{2+} \right]\left[Fe^{3+} \right]^5}{\left[MnO_4^- \right]\left[H^+ \right]^8 \left[Fe^{2+} \right]^5} = 63.5$$

$$\log \frac{\left[Mn^{2+} \right]\left[Fe^{3+} \right]^5}{\left[MnO_4^- \right]\left[H^+ \right]^8 \left[Fe^{2+} \right]^5} = 3 \times 10^{63}$$

$$K = 3 \times 10^{63}$$

It is clear from the large valve of K, (the equilibrium constant) that the reaction will proceed to the completion, the residual ferrous iron concentration being of negligible proposition.

3.4 Types of Redox Titrations

The major types of the redox titration with their titrant are depicted in Table.3.1 as;

Table 3.1: Types of redox titration

S. No.	Type of redox titration	Titrant
1	Permangnatometry	$KMnO_4$
2	Dichromatometry	$K_2Cr_2O_7$
3	Iodimetry	I_2
4	Iodometry	$Na_2S_2O_3$
5	Cerimetry	$Ce(SO_4)_2$
6	Bromatometry	$KBrO_3$
7	Iodatometry	IO_3^-

1. $KMnO_4$ (potassium permanganate) titrations: Potassium permanganate (formula = $KMnO_4$, molecular weight = 158.03) is a strong oxidising agent and is most important compound of manganese in which the oxidation state of the latter is 7+ (Mn^{+7}).

Infact this is the potassium salt of permanganic acid ($HMnO_4$). It is used as anti-infective. The permanganate method is based on reaction of oxidation by the permanganate ion. Oxidation may proceed in acid or in alkaline solution, when $KMnO_4$ acts as an oxidising agent in acid solution;

$$MnO_4^- \xrightarrow{\text{(oxidised to)}} Mn^{2+}$$

Septavelent manganese	Divalent manganese

When $KMnO_4$ is used as a reducing agent in alkaline solution;

$$MnO_4^- \xrightarrow{\text{(Reduced to)}} Mn^{4+}O_2$$

Septavelent manganese	Quadrivalent manganese

No indicator is used for the titrations with permanganate because $KMnO_4$ acts as self indicator. Permanganate solution must be kept in dark places or dark glass because light accelerates decomposition of $KMnO_4$ by reaction:

$$4\ KMnO_4 + 2H_2O \longrightarrow \ \downarrow 4MnO_2 + 4KOH + 3O\uparrow$$

Equivalent Weight of KMnO₄

1. In acidic medium: [H₂SO₄]

$$10\ FeSO_4 + 2KMnO_4 + 8H_2SO_4 \longrightarrow 5\ Fe_2(SO_4)_3 + 2MnSO_4$$
$$+ K_2SO_4 + 8H_2O$$

Ionic form: $5\ Fe^{2+} + MnO_4^- + 8H^+ \rightleftharpoons 5Fe^{3+} + Mn^{2+} + 4H_2O$

Half reaction: $5\ Fe^{2+} \rightleftharpoons 5Fe^{3+} + 5e^-$ \qquad (Oxidation)

$MnO_4^- + 8H^+ + 5e^- \rightleftharpoons Mn^{2+} + 4H_2O$ \qquad (Reduction)

In such a redox reaction permanganate ion is converted into manganese ion by gaining $5e^-$. Therefore,

$$\text{Eq. wt.} = \frac{MW}{\text{Gain of Electrons}} = \frac{158.03}{5} = 31.61 \text{ g}$$

2. In alkaline medium: [KOH]

$$Cr_2(SO_4)_3 + 2KMnO_4 + 8KOH \longrightarrow 2K_2CrO_4 + \downarrow 2MnO_2 +$$
$$2K_2SO_4 + 4H_2O$$

Ionic form: $MnO_4^- + 2H_2O + 3e^- \longrightarrow MnO_2 + 2H_2O$

In this reaction gram equivalent weight of MnO_4 has a different value as:

$$Equivalent\ wt. = \frac{158.03}{3} = 52.68\ g$$

Preparation of 0.1 N KMNO$_4$

$$Eq\ wt. = MW/gain\ of\ electrons = \frac{158.03}{5} = 31.61$$

Weight accurately 31.61 g of $KMnO_4$, dissolve it in 1000 ml of distilled water to give 1 N solution and 3.161 g of $KMnO_4$ in 1000 ml of distilled water to give 0.1 N $KMnO_4$.

Standardization of 0.1N KMnO$_4$ by Oxalic Acid / Na Oxalate

Many primary standards have been proposed for standardization of $KMnO_4$ solutions; they include oxalic acid ($H_2C_2O_4$. $2H_2O$), sodium oxalate ($Na_2C_2O_4$), arsenic trioxide (AS_2O_3), and metallic iron. The most convenient of these are $Na_2C_2O_4$ and $H_2C_2O_4$. $2H_2O$. Both these substances are chemically inert and must correspond exactly to their formulas.

The reaction taking place when these substances are titrated with permanganate is represented by the equations:

$$5\ H_2C_2O_4 + 2\ KMnO_4 + 3H_2SO_4 \longrightarrow K_2SO_4 + 2MnSO_4 + 8H_2O$$
$$+ 10CO_2\uparrow$$

Ionic form: $5\ C_2O_4^{2-} + MnO_4 + 16\ H^+ \rightleftharpoons 2\ Mn^{2+} + 8\ H_2O$
$$+ 10\ CO_2\uparrow$$

Half reaction: $5\ C_2O_4^{2-} \rightleftharpoons 10\ CO_2 + 10\ e^-$ (Oxidation)

$MnO_4^- + 16H^+ + 10e^- \rightleftharpoons Mn^{2+} + 8H_2O$ (Reduction)

Procedure: Pipette out 25 ml of oxalic acid or sodium oxalate ($Na_2C_2O_4$), add 10-15 ml of 2N H_2SO_4 and heat the liquid up to 75-80°C. Titrate with 0.1 N $KMnO_4$. The end point is reached when 1 drop of MnO_4^- colors the whole solution to pink which persists for 30 seconds.

2. Potassium dichromate titration: The dichromate titration method is based on reaction of oxidation by the dichromate ion.

Preparation and Standardization of 0.1 N $K_2Cr_2O_7$

$K_2Cr_2O_7$ is not a powerful oxidising agent as $KMnO_4$. But has several advantages over it;

   (i) It can be obtained pure.

   (ii) The standard solution of exactly known concentration of $K_2Cr_2O_7$ can be prepared by weighing out the pure dry salt and dissolving it in the proper volume of water.

   (iii) They are stable towards light.

   (iv) The aqueous solution of $K_2Cr_2O_7$ is stable indefinitely. It can be used in acid as well as in alkaline solution.

$K_2Cr_2O_7$ is used in determination of iron in iron ores;

$$K_2Cr_2O_7 + 6\,FeCl_2 + 14\,HCl \longrightarrow 2CrCl_3 + 2KCl + FeCl_3$$
$$+ 7H_2O$$
$$Cr_2O_7^- + 6\,Fe^{2+} + 14\,H^+ \longrightarrow 2\,Cr^{3+} + Fe^{3+} + 7H_2O$$

$$\therefore \text{ Therefore Eq. wt of } K_2Cr_2O_7 = \frac{294.6}{6} = 49.03 \text{ g}$$

By dissolving 49.03 g of $K_2Cr_2O_7$ in 1000 ml of distilled water gives 1N solution and by dissolving 4.903 g of $K_2Cr_2O_7$ in 1000 ml of distilled water gives 0.1N solution.

Standardization of $K_2Cr_2O_7$: Using Ammonium Iron (II) Sulphate

Take 50 ml of 0.1 M ferrous ammonium sulphate solution, add 20 ml in H_2SO_4 and add 0.5 ml of N-phenylanthrallic acid of indicator. Titrate the excess of the Iron (II) salt with standard 0.02 M $K_2Cr_2O_7$ until the color changes from green to restore red color.

$$2\,Cr^{3+} + 3\,S_2O_8^{2-} + 7H_2O \longrightarrow CrO_7^- + 6\,HSO_4^- + 8\,H^+$$
$$2\,S_2O_8^{2-} + 2\,H_2O \longrightarrow O_2(g) + Fe^{3+} + 4\,HSO_4^-$$

3. Iodometric and iodimetric titrations

Iodine is a mild oxidising agent. Iodine is reduced according to the half reaction as;

$$I_2(s) + 2e^- \rightleftharpoons 2I^-$$

Iodine   Iodide

A solution of iodine is aqueous iodide and has an intense yellow color to brown color. One drop of 0.05 M iodine solution imports a perceptible pale yellow color to 100 ml of water. In colorless solution, iodine can serve as its own indicator. The test is made much more sensitive by causing a solution of starch as indication. Starch reacts with iodine in the presence of iodide to form an intensely blue-colored complex, which is visible at very low concentration of iodine.

Starch should be added near the equivalence point in iodometric titration because it gives a water insoluble complex with iodine and indicates release of iodine from KI (reducing agent).

Direct iodometric titration termed **iodimetry** refers to titrations with a standard solution of iodine. **Indirect** iodometric titrations method, termed **iodometry** deals with the titrations of Iodine liberated in conical flask reactions.

1. Iodimetry: Standard solutions of Iodine may be prepared from accurately weighing the pure reagent. It is simpler to make up the solution from the reagent grade product and then to standardize it. Iodine is slightly soluble in H_2O, but it forms a soluble tri-iodide ion in solution of iodide.

$$I_2 + I^- \rightleftharpoons I_3^-$$

The use of iodide in the solution both increases the solubility of the iodine and decreases its volatility, thus controlling to the stability of the iodide solution. The arsenic trioxide is oxidised by iodine according to the equation:

$$H_3AsO_3 + I_2 + H_2O \rightleftharpoons HAsO_4^{2-} + 4H^+ + 2I^-$$

The position of the equilibrium depends upon the pH.

2. Iodometry: In iodometry, the formation of iodine takes place as a result of hydrogen iodide (HI), with an oxidising agent. The HI is obtained directly in the reaction flask by the action of dilute HCl or H_2SO_4 on a solution of KI. Free iodine is liberated as a result of the oxidation of KI in acidic solution. The liberated iodine is titrated with standard solution of Sodium thiosulphate ($Na_2S_2O_3$).

$$2 KI + H_2SO_4 \longrightarrow K_2SO_4 + 2HI$$

Potassium iodide   Hydrogen iodide

Starch mucilage acts as an indicator which gives blue color with free Iodine.

$$I_2 + 2Na_2S_2O_3 \longrightarrow 2 NaI + Na_2S_4O_6$$

Sodium thiosulphate   Sodium tetrathionate

Example: Assay of $CuSO_4.5H_2O$ (Copper sulphate)

Assay of $CaOCl_2$ (Chlorinated lime)

Assay of Iodine

I.P.Limit: Iodine contains not less than 99.5% and not more than equivalent of 100.5% of iodine.

Procedure: Weigh accurately iodine (0.5 g) and dissolve in a solution of potassium iodide (1 g) in H_2O (5 ml). Dilute it with water to 25 ml, acidify with acetic acid (1ml) and titrate with 0.1 N sodium thiosulphate till light yellow color is obtained. At this stage, add starch mucilage and the titration is continued till blue color disappears.

$$I_2 + 2Na_2S_2O_3 \longrightarrow 2 NaI + Na_2S_4O_6$$

Sodium thiosulphate   Sodium tetrathionate

Starch is added toward the end of titration, when most of iodine is reacted with sodium thiosulphate as starch mucilage forms stable complex with excess of iodine.

4. Titration of Ceric Ammonium Sulphate

This titration involves the use of ceric salt which is a powerful oxidising agent. Ceric salt have intense yellow color. The oxidising power of the ceric salts depends upon the concentration and the type of acid used in the assay.

e.g., Ce^{+4} (IV) in HNO_3 and $HClO_4$ is stronger oxidising agent (monoprotic)

Ce^{+4} (IV) in H_2SO_4 are weaker oxidising agent (diprotic acid)

The fluorides and phosphate have tendency to interfere with concern ions because they form precipitates with them as ceric fluorides and ceric phosphate. The end point of cerimetric titration is indicated by using redox indicator as; ferroin, diphenyl sulphonate, and N-phenylanthrallic acid.

Advantage:

(1) Stability on boiling

(2) Stable towards light

(3) Ce^{+4} are colorless causes no hindrance in detecting end point.

Sulphuric acid solution of ceric sulphate is stable even at boiling but HCl acid solution is unstable due to its reduction resulting in the liberation of free chlorine.

$$2\,Ce^{+4} + 2Cl^- \rightleftharpoons 3\,Ce^{+3} + Cl_2$$

Preparing 0.1 N $(CeSO_4)_2$: $Ce^{4+} + e \rightleftharpoons Ce^{3+}$

$$(IV) \qquad\qquad (III)$$

Calculating the equivalent weight of ceric sulphate $(CeSO_4)_2$ as;

$$Eq.\ wt = \frac{333.25}{1} = 333.25$$

Therefore by dissolving 333.25 g of ceric sulphate $(CeSO_4)_2$ in 1000 ml of distilled water you can prepare the solution equal to 0.1 N and for 0.1 N solution divide both sides by 10 as;

$$\frac{333.25}{10} \longrightarrow 100\ ml \longrightarrow \frac{1\,N}{10}$$

or 33.325 g in 1000 ml → 0.1 N

Weight out 33 g of pure cerium (IV) sulphate into a 500 ml beaker, add 56 ml of 1:1 mixture of sulphuric acid and H_2O. Then stir with frequent addition of water with gentle warming, until the salt is dissolved. Transfer it to a graduated volumetric flask and when cold, dilute to the mass with distilled H_2O.

Standardization with Mohr's Salt

Principle: $FeSO_4$, the acidic constituent of Mohr's salt $FeSO_4$ $(NH_4)_3\ SO_4.\ 6\ H_2O$ reduces Ce (IV) to Ce (III) itself getting oxidised to $FeSO_4$.

$$Ce^{+4} + Fe^{+2} \longrightarrow Ce^{+3} + Fe^{+3}$$

Procedure: Pipette out 25 ml of ferrous ammonium sulphate solution into a conical flask. Add 25 ml of H_2SO_4 and 2 drops of ferrous indicator. Titrate it against ceric sulphate solution till the orange color changes to blue.

3.5 Indicators Used in Oxidation and Redox Titration

(1) Self indicators: The $KMnO_4$ solution is quite deeply colored and with a slight excess of the reagent ion, titration is easily detected. Thus in titration of oxalic acid, ferrous ammonium sulphate $Fe(NH_4)_2SO_4$ and H_2O_2 with $KMnO_4$ as soon as the reaction is complete and a drop of the latter is in excess, a light pink color is itself developed, indicating the reaction is complete and the end point has reached.

(2) Internal Indicator: This is a substance which reacts in a specific manner with one of the reagent in a titration to exhibit a color. Thus, starch produces deep blue color with iodine and thiocyanate ion produces a red color with Fe^{3+} ion.

(3) External or spot test indicator: There are usually employed when no internal indicator are used, e.g.,

$$K_3Fe(CN)_6 \rightleftharpoons 3K^+ + Fe(CN)_6^{3-}$$

Potassium ferricyanide   Ferricyanide ion

$$2[Fe(CN)_6]^{3+} \rightleftharpoons 3Fe^{2+} + Fe_3[Fe(CN)_6]_2$$

Ferro-ferricyanide (deep blue to green)

(4) Redox indicator: A redox indicator (also called an oxidation-reduction indicator) is an indicator that undergoes a definite color change at a specific electrode potential. Redox indicators are generally of two types:

1. **General:** Varies as a function of E_{cell}.
2. **Specific:** React with a specific chemical species involved in the titration.

1. General: It relies on a color change with Ind_{ox} and Ind_{red} being different colors.

$$In_{Ox} + ne^- \rightleftharpoons In_{Red}$$

A redox indicator exhibits different color in oxidised and reduced forms. Applying the Nernst equation on redox indicator system as;

$$E = E^0_{Ind} + \frac{0.0591}{n} \log \frac{[In_{Ox}]}{[In_{Red}]}$$

In order to see a color change, approximately a 10% conversion from one form to another is needed.

$$\frac{[In_{Red}]}{[In_{Ox}]} = \frac{1}{10} \text{ or } \geq 10$$

Therefore, the range of color change is at $E = E^0_{Ind} \pm 0.0592 / n$. The electrode potential (E) range for the color change of redox indicator depends on the number of electrons involved. e.g.,

if $n = 1$ then the valve for $\Delta E = 0.118V$

$n = 2$ $\qquad\qquad\qquad \Delta E = 0.0592 \text{ V}$

$n = 3$ $\qquad\qquad\qquad \Delta E = 0.0395 \text{ V}$

2. Specific: The example under specific redox indicator includes starch.

$$\text{Starch} + I_3^- \rightleftharpoons \text{Blue complex}$$

It is easy to detect and is profoundly rapid indicator. This helps us to explain why iodine is a common titrant even though it is a weak oxidant. Another common use is to prepare the starch iodine complex as an indicator.

3.6 Theory of Redox Indicators

Every titration does not require an indicator. In some cases, either the reactants or the products are strongly colored and can serve as the indicator. For example, an oxidation-reduction titration using potassium permanganate (pink/purple) as the titrant does not require an indicator.

Diphenylamine is used as redox indicator in dichromate titration for determining Fe^{+2} from $FeCl_2$.

$$K_2Cr_2O_7 + 6 \ FeCl_2 \longrightarrow 2 \ CrCl_3 + 6 \ FeCl_3 + 2 \ KCl$$
$$+ 14 \ HCl \qquad\qquad + 7 \ H_2O$$

In acid solution the reduction of $K_2Cr_2O_7$ may be represented as,

Reduction: $Cr_2O_7^{2-} + 14H^+ + 6 \ e^- \rightleftharpoons 2 \ Cr^{3+} + 7 \ H_2O$

Oxidation: $6 \ Fe^{2+} \rightleftharpoons 6 \ Fe^{3+} + 6e^-$

When all the Fe^{2+} ions are oxidised to Fe^{3+} ions, excess of chromate ions oxidize diphenylamine to diphenyl benzidine. In redox titration, a sharp color change in I_n occurs only if its E^0 lies between standard potential of oxidation reduction system being titrated against each other.

0.76 → E^0 (V) of diphenylamine indicator.

0.77 → E^0 (V) of ferrous ferric system.

+ 0.01 → Difference.

In order to overcome the variation of +0.01, phosphoric acid is added in the solution in order to get sharp color change at the end point.

Table 3.1: *Some commonly used redox indicators.*

Indicator	$E^0(V)$	Color of Ox. form	Color of Red. form
2,2'-Bipyridine	+1.33 V	Colorless	Yellow
Phenylanthranilic acid	+1.08 V	Violet-red	Colorless
Diphenylamine	+0.76 V	Violet	Colorless
Sodium diphenylamine sulfonate	+0.84 V	Red-violet	Colorless
Diphenylbenzidine	+0.76 V	Violet	Colorless

3.7 Oxidation Reduction Curves

In acid-base titrations titration curves are plotted in terms of pH or pOH versus the concentration of standard while in redox titrations the titration curves are plotted in terms of **cell potential (E_{cell})** versus the **percent titration** of the standard. For each redox titration curve, there are five significant regions shown in (Fig. 3.2).

1. The start: 0% titration. It is the point at which titration starts.

2. Buffering regions: > 0%, < equivalence point. It is a region where the reducing agent takes small amount of time to lose all the electrons and subsequently the electrons are gained by an oxidising agent to reach the equivalence point.

3. The equivalence point: It is the region where the percentage of oxidised and reduced form are equivalent to each other. At this point there is a sharp increase in curve till the end point is reached.

4. Inflection point: A point on a curve at which tangent crosses the curve itself or a point on a curve at which the curvature changes sign. The curve changes from being concave upwards (positive curvature) to concave downwards (negative curvature).

5. Overtitration: It is the region showing the constant curve or potential and color showing by the indicator will be deep at this significant region.

The titration curve in redox reactions can be explained by taking the example of titration between Fe^{2+} and Ce^{4+}. Between 0% and 100% titration, we can use the Nernst equation for Fe^{2+}/e^{3+}:

$$E_{Fe} = 0.771 - 0.0592 \log Fe^{2+}/Fe^{3+}$$

We can simplify our calculations by using the % titration

$$E_{Fe} = 0.771 - 0.0592 \log [\%Fe^{2+}]/[\% Fe^{3+}]$$

At greater than 100% titration, predominate change is that Ce^{4+} is being added and diluted into a solution of Ce^{3+}. All Fe^{2+} has been converted to Fe^{3+} and no longer figures into the calculations. The amounts of Ce^{3+} and Ce^{4+} and the total volume of the system are kept in track.

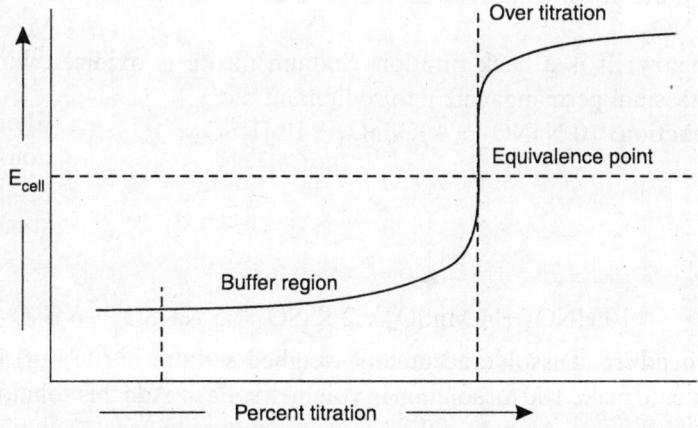

Fig. 3.2: *Redox titration curve showing four significant regions*

3.8 Important Assay of the Oxidation Reduction Titrations

1. Assay of Ferrous Sulphate (FeSO$_4$. 7H$_2$O)

IP limit: Ferrous sulphate contains not less than 98% and not more than 105% of FeSO$_4$.7 H$_2$O.

Theory: Ferrous sulphate is oxidised by potassium permanganate (KMnO$_4$) into the ferric sulphate [Fe^{3+}]. When whole ferrous sulphate is consumed, a drop of potassium permanganate (KMnO$_4$) will give the pink color at the end point.

Reaction:

$$10\ FeSO_4 + 2\ KMnO_4 + 8\ H_2SO_4 \longrightarrow 5\ Fe_2(SO_4)_3 + K_2SO_4 + 2\ MnSO_4 + 8\ H_2O$$

Procedure: Weigh accurately 1g of FeSO$_4$. Dissolve it in 20 ml dilute solution of H$_2$SO$_4$ and titrate the required solution with 0.1N KMnO$_4$. Continue titration till pink color persists for 30 seconds.

Eq. factor: Each 1 ml of 0.1N KMO$_4$ is equivalent to 0.0278 g of FeSO$_4$.7H$_2$O.

$$\% \text{ purity} = \frac{\text{Vol. of } 0.1\ N\ KMnO_4\text{ used} \times \text{Eq. factor}}{\text{Weight of FeSO}_4.7\ H_2O} \times 100$$

2. Assay of Sodium Nitrite (NaNO$_2$)

IP limit: It contains not less than 98% and not more than 105% of NaNO$_2$.

Theory: It is a back titration. Sodium nitrite is oxidised with potassium permanganate into sodium nitrate.

Reaction: $10\ NaNO_2 + 4\ KMnO_4 + 12\ H_2SO_4$

$$\downarrow$$

$$10\ HNO_3 + 4\ MnSO_4 + 2\ K_2SO_4 + 5\ Na_2SO_4 + 6\ H_2O$$

Procedure: Dissolve accurately weighed sodium nitrite (1g) in water to make 100 ml solution in volumetric flask. Add this solution (10 ml) into a mixture of 0.1 N potassium permanganate solution (50 ml), sulfuric acid (5 ml) and water (100 ml). Warm the mixture

up to 40 °C, add 0.1 N oxalic acid (25 ml). Heat the mixture to 60 °C on a water bath and titrate with 0.1 N potassium permanganate solution till pink color persists for 30 seconds after shaking.
Factor: Each ml 0.1 N $KMnO_4$ is equivalent to 0.00345 g of $NaNO_2$.

3. Assay of Hydrogen Peroxide (H_2O_2)

IP limit: It contains not less than 5% w/v and not more than 7% w/v of H_2O_2 corresponding to 20 volume strength.

Theory: Hydrogen peroxide has both oxidising and reducing properties, but if titrated against an acidified potassium permanganate it acts as a reducing agent .When hydrogen peroxide is reacted with potassium permanganate it is oxidised into oxygen. High concentration of the acid is used to prevent the formation of manganese dioxide which may cause decomposition of hydrogen peroxide.

The reaction of assay is given as:

$$5\,H_2O_2 + 2\,KMnO_4 \longrightarrow 5\,O_2\uparrow + 2\,MnSO_4 + K_2SO_4$$
$$+ 3\,H_2SO_4 \qquad\qquad + 8H_2O$$

Procedure: Dilute hydrogen peroxide (10 to 25 ml) with water, add 5 N sulphuric acid (5 ml) and titrate with 0.1 N potassium permanganate solution to a permanent pink end point.

Factor: Each ml 0.1 N $KMnO_4$ is equivalent to 0.01701 g of H_2O_2.

4. Assay of Copper Sulphate ($CuSO_4 . 5 H_2O$)

IP limit: It contains not less than 98.5% and not more than the equivalent of 101% of $CuSO_4 . 5H_2O$.

Theory: Copper sulphate is assayed by iodometric method. Reducing agent potassium iodide (KI) is added in the presence of acetic acid to form cupric iodide. Acetic acid is added to form a weakly acidic solution. Cupric iodide is unstable and decomposes it cuprous iodide and iodine. The liberated iodine is titrated with sodium thiosulphate till the solution becomes yellow. Most of the liberated iodine is reacted with sodium thiosulphate. Little amount is left (indicated by yellow color). Starch mucilage is added towards the end because it forms stable complex with excess of iodine.

$$2\,CuSO_4 + 4\,KI \longrightarrow 2\,CuI_2 + 2\,K_2SO_4$$

$$\underset{\text{Cupric iodide}}{2\,CuI_2} \longrightarrow \underset{\text{Cuprous iodide}}{Cu_2I_2} + I_2$$

$$I_2 + 2\,Na_2S_4O_6 \longrightarrow 2\,Na_2S_4O_6 + 2\,NaI$$

The decomposition of cupric iodide into cuprous iodide and iodine is reversible, hence to make quantitative, potassium thiocyanate is added which reacts with the reaction product, cuprous iodide, to form cuprous thiocyanate.

$$\underset{\text{Cuprous iodide}}{Cu_2I_2} + KCNS \longrightarrow \underset{\text{Cuprous thiocyanate}}{CuCNS} + 2\,KI$$

Procedure: Weight accurately copper sulphate (1g), dissolve in water (50 ml), add potassium iodide (3 g) and acetic acid (5 ml) and titrate the liberated iodine with 0.1 N sodium thiosulphate till light yellow color is obtained. At this stage starch mucilage and potassium thiocyanate (2 g) are added and the titration is continued until blue color disappears and does not return after several minutes.
Factor: Each ml of 0.1 N $Na_2S_2O_3$ is equivalent to 0.02497 g of $CuSO_4 \cdot 5H_2O$.

EXERCISES

---

1. Calculate equivalent weight of potassium permanganate ($KMnO_4$) in acidic and alkaline medium.
2. Write preparation and standardization of 0.1 N of potassium permanganate ($KMnO_4$). Give assay of ferrous sulphate ($FeSO_4$).
3. Explain oxidation and reduction titration in detail.
4. Write briefly about the iodometric and iodimetric titrations. Give examples.
5. Why starch should be added near the equivalence point in iodimetric titrations?
6. Write briefly about the titrations with ceric salts in redoximetry. Give examples.
7. Write preparation and standardization of 0.1 N of potassium dichromate ($K_2Cr_2O_7$).

8. Explain oxidation and reduction curve in detail.

9. Write briefly about the indicators used in oxidation and reduction titrations. Give Examples.

10. What do you understand by oxidation and reduction?

11. Explain redox titrations with examples.

12. Calculate the equivalent weight of some reducing agents.

13. Give the theory of the redox indicators. Mention there types also.

14. Explain the stability of potassium permanganate ($KMnO_4$) solution and how it can be standardized.

15. What is the difference between iodometry and iodimetry? Give examples of the titrations involving these principles.

16. Explain the reaction in which iodine is liberated in iodometric titrations.

17. What are the different types of the titrations based on the concept of oxidation and reduction? Explain with examples.

18. Explain Nernst equation for electrode potential?

19. Define equivalent weight of an oxidising and a reducing agent.

20. Write the titrations involving potassium permanganate and potassium dichromate.

21. Write the assay procedure of copper sulphate in detail.

22. Write preparation and standardization of 0.1 N of I_2 solutions.

23. Write a detail about the calculation of standard electrode potential.

24. Write the theory and procedure of sodium nitrite and hydrogen peroxide.

25. Mention the four significant regions of the redox curves and show them graphically?

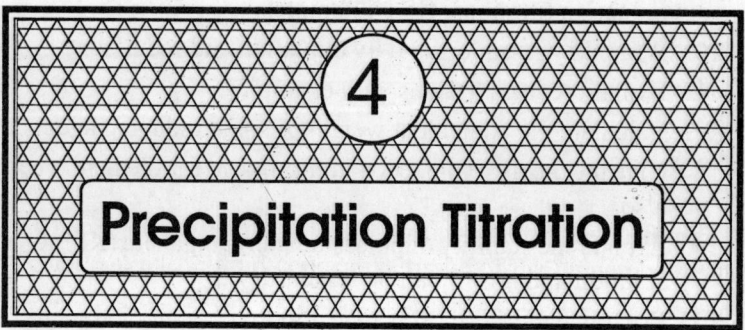

4

Precipitation Titration

Titration is a process by which the concentration of an unknown substance or sample in a solution is determined by adding measured amounts of a standard solution that reacts with the unknown sample. Then the concentration of the unknown substance can be calculated using the stoichiometry of the reaction and the number of moles of standard solution needed to reach the so called end point.

Precipitation titrations are based upon reactions that yield ionic compounds of limited solubility. The most important precipitating reagent is silver nitrate. Titrimetric methods based upon silver nitrate are sometimes termed as argentometric methods. Potassium chromate can serve as an end point indicator for the argentometric determination of chloride, bromide and cyanide ions by reacting with silver ions to form a brick-red silver chromate precipitate in the equivalence point region.

Precipitation

Precipitation means 'formation of precipitate or insoluble complex' and precipitation titration comprises a class of reactions that requires a formation of insoluble precipitate provided that the end point at which the precipitation is complete can be determined. In precipitation titrations, the formation of insoluble precipitate occurs due to some reagent called precipitating reagent possessing the precipitating ions, e.g.,

1. NH_4CNS (ammonium thiocyanate) and precipitating ion is CNS^- (thiocyanate ion).

2. KCNS (potassium thiocyanate) and precipitating ion is CNS^- (thiocyanate ion).

3. $AgNO_3$ (silver nitrate) and precipitating ion is Ag^+ (silver ion).

4.1 Argentometric Titrations

The precipitation process in titrimetric analysis using silver nitrate $(AgNO_3)$ as a reagent is called argentometric titrations. Therefore, "The part of titrimetric analysis in which precipitation of compound occurs by titrating against the standard silver nitrate $(AgNO_3)$ solution is called argentometric titration", e.g., when a solution of sodium chloride (NaCl) is added to solution of silver nitrate $(AgNO_3)$, a white precipitate of silver chloride (AgCl) is formed (chloride limit test).

$$AgNO_3 \ + \ NaCl \ \longrightarrow \ AgCl\downarrow \ + \ NaNO_3$$

Silver nitrate   Silver chloride   Sodium nitrate
           (white precipitate)

Principle: The main principle of the precipitation titrations is that the quantity of the added precipitating reagent or precipitant is equivalent to the substance being precipitated.

Types of Argentometric Titrations

(1) Direct titration Method: (Mohr's Method)

The substance in solution is directly titrated with a titrant or precipitant and the end point in the precipitation is determined by the use of internal indicator. E.g., assay of sodium chloride (NaCl):

$$NaCl \ + \ H_2O \ \longrightarrow \ K_2CrO_4 \ [\text{Potassium chromate}$$

Sodium chloride   (indicator)]

$$\xrightarrow{\text{add}} \ \text{Titrate against 0.1 AgNO3 till}$$

brick red color is obtained

2. Indirect Titration Method or Back Titration: (Volhard's Method)

The excess of silver nitrate ($AgNO_3$) is added to the solution of halide acidified with nitric acid. The unreacted silver nitrate ($AgNO_3$) is treated against standard ammonium thiocyanate (NH_4CNS) solution using ferric salt (Ferric NH_4^+ SO_4^{2-}) as an indicator, e.g., assay of NH_4Cl:

$NH_4Cl + H_2O$ + Nitric acid + Nitrobenzene + $AgNO_3$ (excess)

⟶ Shake vigorously for one minute and add ferric salt indicator

⟶ Titrate with 0.1N NH_4SCN till reddish brown color.

4.2 Preparation and Standardization of 0.1 N AgNO₃ Solution

I.P.Limit: Silver nitrate contains not less than 99.9% and not more than 100% of $AgNO_3$.

Preparation: The 0.1 N solution of silver nitrate can be prepared by dissolving 16.98 g of silver nitrate in water and adjusting the volume up to 1000 ml.

Standardization: A silver nitrate solution may be standardized against a standard solution of sodium chloride using potassium chromate as an indicator (Mohr's method). The standardization depends upon the reactions expressed as follows:

$$AgNO_3 + NaCl \longrightarrow AgCl + NaNO_3$$

Silver nitrate   Sodium chloride   Silver chloride   Sodium nitrate

$AgNO3 = NaCl = H$

169.8 g AgNO3 = 58.45 g NaCl = 1000 ml N

Therefore, 0.01698 g AgNO3 = 0.005845 g NaCl = 1 ml 0.1 N AgNO3.

4.3 Solubility Product

The process of precipitation titration is completely based on the concept of solubility product. Let us consider a dissociation of slightly soluble salt AB. In solution it will exist in equilibrium with its dissociation ions as:

$$AB \rightleftharpoons A^+ + B^-$$

Applying law of Mass action:

$$K = \frac{[A^+].[B^-]}{[AB]}$$

The concentration of the AB in the solution remains constant in the presence of undissolved AB, i.e.,

$$K_{SP} = \frac{[A^+].[B^-]}{[AB]} \Rightarrow K_{SP} = [A^+][B^-]$$

Where K_{SP} is unchanged at constant temperature and is called solubility product of salt (AB) and is defined as the maximum product of the concentration of its constituent ions in its solution.

$[A^+]$ and $[B^-]$ = Concentration of constituent ions in saturated solution

If the ionic product or concentration is greater (>) than $K_{SP} \rightarrow$ precipitation will occur.

If the ionic product or concentration is lesser (<) than $K_{SP} \rightarrow$ precipitation do not occur.

If ionic concentration = K_{SP} (solution remains saturated),

Therefore lesser the solubility product, easier will be the precipitation.

The silver halide e.g. silver chloride (AgCl), silver bromide (AgBr) and silver iodide (AgI) are easily precipitated due to very small value of K_{SP}.

$$AgCl \longrightarrow 1.8 \times 10^{-10}$$
$$AgBr \longrightarrow 5.2 \times 10^{-13}$$
$$AgI \longrightarrow 8.3 \times 10^{-17}$$

Based on solubility product if excess Ag^+ ions are added to the saturated solution of silver chloride (AgCl) in H_2O, the ionic product of $[Ag^+][Cl^-]$ is exceeded and consequently some silver chloride (AgCl) will be precipitated. The phenomenon of precipitating ion is also described by the solubility product.

Importance of Solubility Product

The great value of the solubility product is that it permits the calculation of one of the ion concentrations if the other is known.

In the pure saturated solution the situation is even simpler because the reaction stoichiometry provides a relationship between the ion concentrations. Thus in a solution of the salt BA, we can write $[B^+] = [A^-]$, because each molecule of BA that dissolves produces one B^+ ion and one A^- ion.

4.4 Fundamentals of Precipitation Titration

Following conditions must be satisfied by a precipitation reaction to act as a titrimetric analysis:

1. The rate of the reaction between the precipitant and the analyte or the substance to be precipitated must be fast.

2. The reaction between the analyte and the reagent should proceed according to a definite stiochoimetric relationship. For example in the reaction of silver nitrate ($AgNO_3$) and potassium thiocyanate (KCNS):

$$AgNO_3 \;+\; KCNS \longrightarrow AgCNS\downarrow \;+\; KNO_3$$

(169.89)	(97.18)	(165.96)	(101.11 g)
(Analyte)	(Precipitant)	(Precipitate)	

169.89 g silver nitrate ($AgNO_3$) reacts with 97.18 g of potassium thiocyanate (KCNS) to gives 165.96 g of silver thiocyanate (AgCNS) and 101.11 g of potassium nitrate (KNO_3).

3. A suitable indicator should be available to locate the end point of the titration.

4. The end point should be well defined.

4.5 Theory and Curve of Argentometry

To understand the theory and curve of precipitation titrations, let us consider the titration of 50.0 ml of 0.1M silver chloride (NaCl) against 0.1 M silver nitrate ($AgNO_3$).The titration is started and the silver nitrate ($AgNO_3$) solution is gradually added from the burette. There is not much increase in concentration of ionic products of silver [Ag]. But on continuing the process, the point is reached when concentration of ionic product exceeds the K_{SP} and consequently some silver chloride (AgCl) will be precipitated.

Therefore, there is sudden rise in Cl^- concentration. On adding the silver nitrate ($AgNO_3$) after the end point, sudden rise continues as soon as the curve becomes flat. Thus, it is possible to calculate chloride (Cl^-) concentration at different stages. If the volume of silver nitrate ($AgNO_3$) added is plotted against different chloride ion concentration (Cl^-), the titration curve is similar to that obtained for acid/base or redox titration (Fig. 4.1).

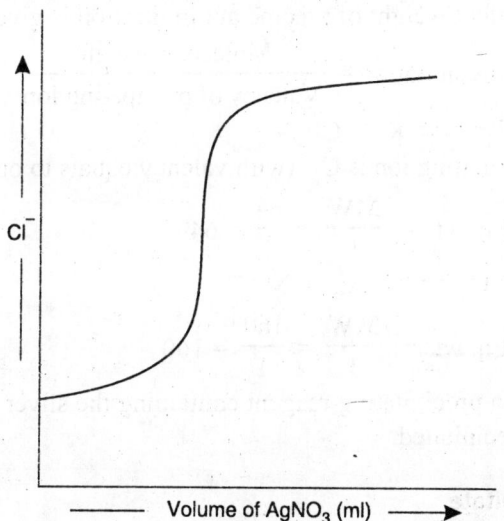

Fig. 4.1: *Titration of silver nitrate ($AgNO_3$) against sodium chloride (NaCl)*

To Achieve the Accurate Precipitation Titration

1. The concentration of analyte and precipitant should be greater and the solution should not be very dilute. Greater concentration means lesser solubility of the precipitate and greater accuracy in location of end point. Smaller K_{SP} means greater value of equilibrium constant for precipitation reaction.

2. The solubility product of the precipitate should be very small, because precipitation occurs only if the ionic product of solution exceeds the solubility product of the respective salt.

3. Based on solubility product, if excess Ag^+ ions are added to the saturated solution of silver chloride (AgCl) in H_2O, the ionic product of $[Ag^+]$ $[Cl^-]$ is exceeded and consequently some silver chloride (AgCl) will be precipitated.

4.6 Equivalent Weight in Precipitation Titrations

The equivalent weight of precipetant in titration is given by:

$$\text{Eq. wt. of precipitation} = \frac{\text{Molecular weight}}{\text{Valency of precipating ion}}$$

1. $KCl \rightleftharpoons K^+ + Cl^-$

Here precipitating ion is Cl^- (with valency equals to one). Thus,

$$\text{Eq. wt.} = \frac{MW}{1} = \frac{64}{1} = 64$$

2. $AgNO_3 \rightleftharpoons Ag^+ + NO_3^-$

$$\text{Eq. wt.} = \frac{MW}{1} = \frac{160}{1} = 160$$

$AgNO_3$ is a precipitating reagent containing the silver ion which is to be precipitated.

4.7 Precipitate

It is a whitish curdy flake like floccules formed in the solution due to addition of precipitating agents e.g. silver nitrate ($AgNO_3$) or ammonium thiocyanate (NH_4SCN) or potassium thiocyanate (KSCN). Precipitate is obtained by adding suitable precipitating agent or reagent in excess from outside to given solution.
Precipitate are of two types:

1. Colloidal precipitate	2. Crystalline precipitate
1. Particle range: 10-2000Å	1. Size greater than 2000 °A
2. Cannot be retained by ordinary and filter paper due to small size	2. They are easily filtered pure

Characteristics of Precipitate

1. It must be highly insoluble.
2. The precipitate should be filterable.
3. It should be of high purity.

4.8 Factors Afecting the Solubility of Precipitate

Factors affecting the solubility of the precipitate includes:

1. Effect of acidity of solution: Let us take the dissociation of sodium chloride (NaCl) as:

$$NaCl \longrightarrow Na^+ + Cl^-$$

Now if the acid solution is added to the soluble salt, again a common ion effect will be experienced;

$$HCl \longrightarrow H^+ + \boxed{Cl^-}$$
$$NaCl \longrightarrow Na^+ + \boxed{Cl^-}$$

$\Bigg\}$ Common ion

Therefore, there will a decrease in solubility of sodium chloride (NaCl) or dissociation of sodium chloride (NaCl).

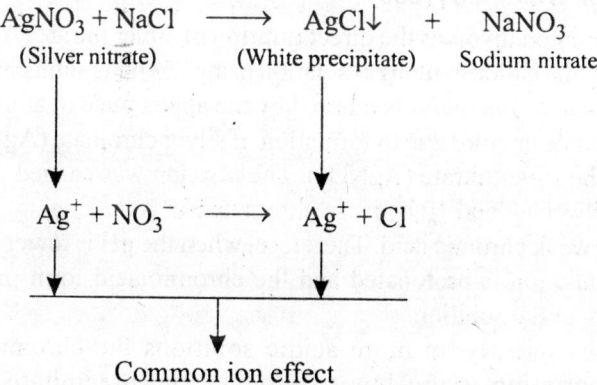

$$AgNO_3 + NaCl \longrightarrow AgCl\downarrow + NaNO_3$$

(Silver nitrate)   (White precipitate)   Sodium nitrate

$$Ag^+ + NO_3^- \longrightarrow Ag^+ + Cl$$

Common ion effect

2. Common ion effect: Increase in the common ion concentration shifts the equilibrium towards the left resulting minimum dissociation of salt from which they are produced.

3. Effect of temperature: The solubility of the precipitate increases with an increase in the temperature of reaction medium. For example, in case of silver chloride and barium sulphate variations are shown as:

Compound		Temperature	
		10°C	100°C
Solubility of AgCl (Ag^+)	$\longrightarrow$	1.72	21.1 mg/lt
Solubility of $BaSO_4$ (Ba^{2+})	$\longrightarrow$	2.2	3.9 mg/lt

According to the Hardy-Schulz rule higher the valency of precipitating ion, the greater is its precipitating power, therefore, $Al^{3+} > Ba^{2+} > Ag^+$. Therefore aluminium ion will precipitate more radially than silver ion.

4. Effect of solvent: Most of the precipitates are inorganic solids showing a polar nature. These are soluble in polar solvents (like water and alcohol) and insoluble in non-polar solvent (like benzene, solvent ether).

4.9 Types of Argentometric Titrations

Depending upon the type of indicator involved in the reaction, there are three types of argentometric titrations (Table 4.1).

1. Mohr's Method (1856)

This method involves the direct titration of silver nitrate ($AgNO_3$) against the halide in **neutral** solution using 2% potassium chromate as indicator. End point is marked by the appearance of a brick red precipitate or color due to formation of silver chromate (Ag_2CrO_4) with the silver nitrate ($AgNO_3$). The titration was carried out at a pH between 7 and 10 because chromate ion is the conjugate base of the weak chromic acid. Therefore, when the pH is lower than 7, chromate ion is protonated and the chromic acid form predominately in the solution.

Consequently, in more acidic solutions the chromate ion concentration is too low to produce the precipitate at the equivalence point. If the pH is above 10, brownish silver hydroxide forms and masks the end point. A suitable pH was achieved by saturating the analyte solution with sodium hydrogen carbonate.

When $AgNO_3$ solution from burette is added to the titration flask containing NaCl and indicator, following reaction occurs:

$$KCrO_4 \rightleftharpoons 2K^+ + CrO_4^{2-}$$

$$NaCl \rightleftharpoons Na^+ + Cl^- \text{ (Ionization in titration flask)}$$

$$Ag^+ + Cl^- \longrightarrow AgCl\downarrow \text{ (White precipitate)}$$

$$2Ag^+ + CrO_4^{2-} \longrightarrow Ag_2CrO_4 \text{ (Brick red color)}$$

Mohr's method is based on solubility product of silver chloride (AgCl) and silver chromate (Ag_2CrO_4).

$$S_P \text{ of AgCl} = 1.2 \times 10^{-12}$$
$$S_P \text{ of Ag}_2\text{CrO}_4 = 8.3 \times 10^{-3}$$

(Less solubility product $\longrightarrow$ Better precipitation)

Hence so long as there is any chloride left in the solution, Ag_2CrO_4 is formed. The Ag_2CrO_4 formed will be changed to AgCl immediately with corresponding halide.

$$Ag_2CrO_4 + 2Cl^- \longrightarrow 2AgCl\downarrow + CrO_4^{2-}$$

Silver chromate   Silver chloride

At the end point, when whole of the chloride has been used up, the Ag_2CrO_4 is formed giving brick red color or precipitate.

Limitations

(i) Silver chromate (Ag_2CrO_4) is soluble in acid solution thus the solution to be titrated should be neutral.

(ii) This method is not suitable for iodides, because of the same color of precipitated silver iodide (AgI) and potassium chromate indicator, i.e., yellow.

***Table 4.1:** Types of argentometric titrations*

	Method/type	Indicator used	Assay	Color change
1.	Mohr's method or direct argentometric method (1856)	2% solution of potassium chromate	NaCl	Yellow Brick red
2.	Volhard's method or indirect Argentometric method (1874)	Ferric ammonium sulphate or ferric salt	NH_4Cl	Reddish brown
3.	Fajan's method (1924)	Adsorption indicator 0.1% fluorescein (Dichlorofluorocein)	NaCl/ KCl	Yellowish pink

2. Volhard's method: (Indirect method or residual titrations). This method was given by Vohlard in 1874. In this method the excess of silver nitrate ($AgNO_3$) is added to the solution of halide acidified with nitric acid. The unreacted silver nitrate ($AgNO_3$) is treated against standard ammonium thiocyanate (NH_4SCN) solution using ferric salt as indicator, e.g., assay of ammonium chloride (NH_4Cl):

NH_4Cl + H_2O + Nitric acid + Nitrobenzene + $AgNO_3$ (excess) $\longrightarrow$ Shake vigorously for one minute and add ferric salt indicator $\longrightarrow$ Titrate with 0.1N ammonium thiocyanate (NH_4SCN) till reddish brown color is obtained.

When standard solution as NH_4SCN is added to a solution of silver salt a precipitate of silver thiocyanate (AgCNS) continues to be formed till the Ag^+ ions are not completely precipitated.

$$Ag^+ + CNS^- \longrightarrow AgCNS\downarrow$$
Silver thiocyanate

The addition of further drop of thiocyanate reacts with the ferric ions to form a reddish brown ferric thiocyanate complex.

$$Fe^{3+} + 3CNS^- \longrightarrow Fe(CNS)_3$$
Red/reddish brown

When the end point is approached, the solution of silver thiocyanate (AgCNS) should be vigorously agitated because a large amount of the Ag^+ ions are absorbed on the surface of AgCNS precipitate which gets removed only very slowly when thiocyanate is added.

Applications: It is employed in the determination of iodides, chlorides and thiocyanate ions.

3. Fajan's Method of Precipitation Titrations

This method was given by K. Fajan in 1924. The method employs adsorption indicators for the detection of end point in precipitation titrations.

Principle: The principle of Fajan's method of precipitation titration is based on the fact that, at the end point, the indicator gets adsorbed by the precipitate resulting in a substance of different color.

Indicators Used in Fajan's Method of Precipitation Titrations

Commonly used indicators in Fajan's method for the titration of halides and isocyanates against silver nitrate are:

1. Fluorescein.
2. Dichlorofluorocein (Mixed).
3. Eosin (Tetrabromofluorescein).
4. Erythrosine (Tetraiodofluorescein) (Fig. 4.2).

Choice of Suitable Adsorption Indicator

1. The indicator ion (fluorescinate ion) must be an opposite charge to the ion of precipitating agent.
2. It should be strongly absorbed immediately after the end point.
3. The indicator should not be adsorbed before the precipitate formation.

4.10 Principle of Adsorption Indicator

The principle of adsorption indicator is based upon the phenomenon of **adsorption**. The phenomenon of concentration of molecules of gas or liquid at a solid surface is termed as adsorption. The substance that concentrates at the surface is called an **adsorbate** and the solid surface on which concentrations occurs is known as **adsorbent**, e.g., silver nitrate ($AgNO_3$) is titrated against sodium chloride (NaCl) solution.

In solution the ions present are;

$$NaCl \longrightarrow Na^+ + Cl^- \text{ (In flask)},$$

$$AgNO_3 \rightleftharpoons Ag^+ + NO_3^- \text{ [In burette]}$$

$$\underset{\text{Silver nitrate}}{AgNO_3} + NaCl \longrightarrow \underset{\text{White precipitate}}{AgCl^-} + \underset{\text{sodium nitrate}}{NaNO_3}$$

The precipitate of silver chloride (AgCl) adsorbs chloride ion (Cl^-) to form a primary adsorbed layer. It will hold secondary adsorbed positively charged ions as Na^+ from solution present in the flask. At end point Ag^+ ions are added from the burette which are not primary adsorbed and oppositively charged NO_3^- ions will form the secondary adsorbed layer. Now on the surface of first traces of Ag^+ ions the modified fluorescinate ions of indicator gets adsorbed.

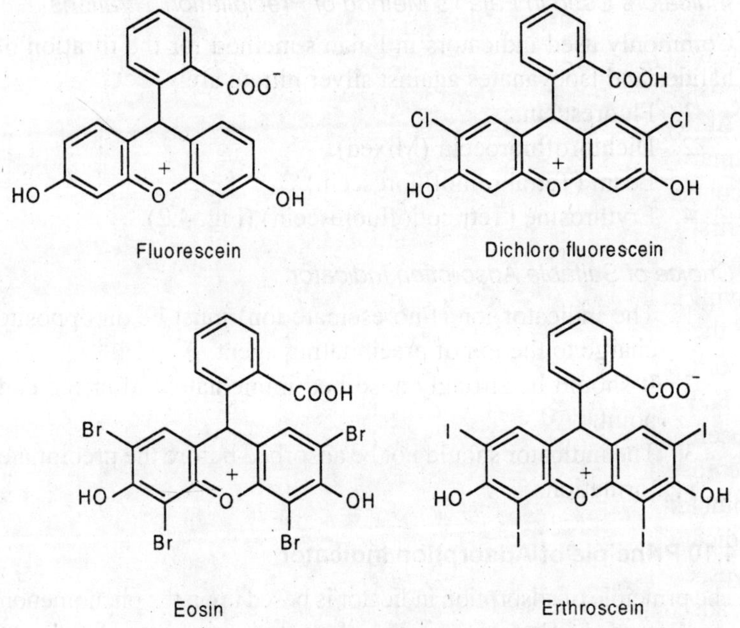

Fluorescein

Dichloro fluorescein

Eosin

Erthroscein

Fig. 4.2: *Indicators used in Fajan's method*

Table 4.2: *Common precipitation indicators*

Indicator	Use	Experimental conditions	Color change at end-point
1. Fluorescein	Halides, e.g., I^-, Cl^-, Br^- with Ag^+.	Neutral or weakly basic solution	Yellow green - Pink
2. Tetrazine	Ag^+ with I^- or SCN-excess Ag+ on back titration, i.e., I^-.	Back titration	Colorless- Green
3. Dichloro-fluorocein	Cl^-, Br^- with Ag^+	PH range 4.4–7.0	Yellow green- Red

4.11 Theory of Adsorption Indicators

The theory is based on reaction of sodium chloride added to silver nitrate ($AgNO_3$) solution. The reaction leads to the formation of silver chloride precipitate ($AgCl\downarrow$). The precipitate absorbs Cl^- ions from the solution, now Cl^- ions will hold secondary absorbed oppositively charged ions as (Na^+) from NaCl in the solution.

At the end point, Ag^+ ions which are present in solution are not primarily adsorbed and oppositively charged NO_3^- ions will form secondary adsorbed layer. It is immediately adsorbed on the surface of first traces of excess of Ag^+ ions to form pink color. After adding the Na^+ salts of fluorescein as indicator, the fluorescinate ions having more adsorption capacity than nitrate ions (NO_3^-) adsorbs on the surface of first traces of excess of Ag^+ ions to form pink color (Fig. 4.3).

K. Fajan, through his studies on nature of adsorption, introduced a useful type of indicator for precipitation titrations. Such indicators are adsorbed on the surface of the precipitate at the equivalence point and this adsorption is accompanied by a color change. These indicators are either acid dyes, e.g., fluorescein and eosin or basic dyes, e.g., rhodamine series. The property of a colloidal precipitate to adsorb its own ions, which are in excess, is used in the case. When a sodium chloride solution is titrated with silver nitrate, the silver chloride precipitate will adsorb chloride ions which are initially in excess. Thus, the chloride ions from the primary adsorbed layer, which in turn will hold the secondary adsorbed layer of oppositely charged Na^+ ions. Immediately after the equivalence point, Ag^+ ions are in excess and hence silver chloride ions now adsorb Ag^+ ions as primary adsorbed layer and NO_3^- as secondary adsorbed layer. Now, if the sodium salt of fluorescein is also present in the solution then the negatively charged fluorescein ions would be adsorbed instead of NO_3^- as secondary adsorbed layers and this adsorption occurs along with a change to pink color due to formation of a pink colored complex of Ag^+ and modified florescence ions. The difference between the Mohr's and Fajan's method are depicted in Table 4.3.

Factors affecting the absorption endpoint:
1. Intensity of color
2. Indicator concentration
3. Precipitate surface area
4. Displacement of primary adsorbed ion

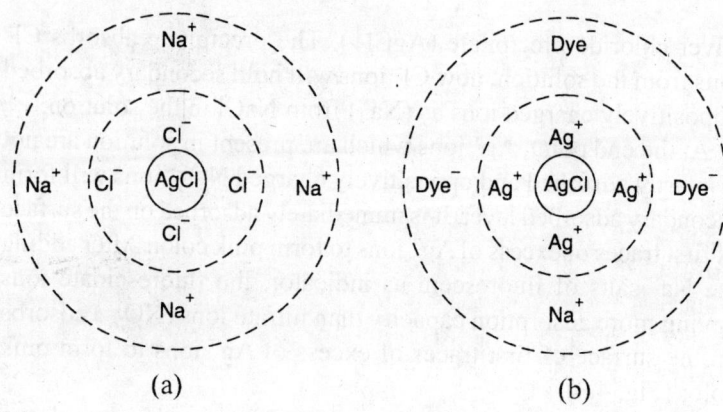

Fig. 4.3: *(a) AgCl precipitated in presence of excess of Cl⁻*
(b) AgCl precipitated in presence of excess of Ag⁺

Precipitate formation titrations curves: As with other types of reactions, the formation of a precipitate can be used as the basis of the titration (Fig. 4.4).

$$\text{Analyte} + \text{Precipitant} \longrightarrow \text{Precipitate}$$

The approach assumes that under the experimental conditions used, the product is virtually insoluble. In determination of Cl⁻ by titration with Ag^+ we have,

$$Ag^+ + Cl^- \longrightarrow AgCl$$

We will assume that both our samples and titrant are 0.1000 M solutions and we will take 50.00 ml of sample for the titration. As soon as addition of Ag^+ is started, silver chloride (AgCl) begins to form.

Based on $K_{sp\ AgCl} = 1.8 \times 10^{-10}$ and $K_{sp\ AgCl}$ is also = $[Ag^+]$ $[Cl^-]$. In this region virtually all $[Ag^+]$ will precipitate as silver chloride (AgCl) and $[Cl^-]$ content can be determined by calculating the amount of AgCl that has precipitated.

Prior to start the titration no chloride has been added to the titrations so calculations are pretty straight forward.

$$[Cl^-] = 0.1000 \text{ M}$$

We need to convert it to the p scale for use in our titration curve.

$$pCl = -\log [Cl^-] = 1.000M$$

$$[Cl^-] = \frac{\text{Starting moles } Cl^- - \text{Moles AgCl precipitated}}{\text{Volume of solution in litres (v)}}$$

Since the quantities are small and we will be using ml quantities of titrants, it is best to use mmoles.

Starting mmoles $[Cl^-] = 50.0$ ml $\times 0.1000$ M
$$= 5.000 \text{mmol}$$

After adding of 5 ml Ag^+
Solution volume = 55ml

$Mmol_{AgCl}$ formed = 5ml $\times 0.1000$M Ag^+
$$= 0.5 \text{ mmoles AgCl}$$

$$[Cl^-] = \frac{\text{Starting moles } Cl^- - \text{Moles AgCl precipitated}}{\text{Volume of solution in litres (v)}}$$

$$[Cl^-] = \frac{5.000 \text{ nmol} - 5 \text{ nmoles}}{55 \text{ ml}}$$

$$= 0.08181 \text{ M}$$

We can also calculate the $[Ag^+]$ using our K_{sp} expression:

$$[Ag^+] = K_{sp} / [Cl^-] = 1.8 \times 10^{-10}/0.08181 \text{ M}$$

$$= 2.20 \times 10^{-9}$$

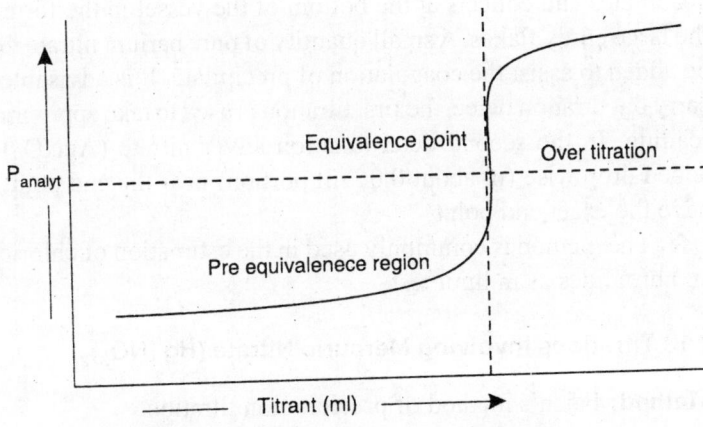

Fig. 4.4: Precipitate formation titrations curve

Finally, we need to convert to p valves.

$$pCl = -\log 0.08181 = \mathbf{1.09}$$
$$pAg = -\log 2.20 \times 10^{-9} = \mathbf{8.66}$$

4.12 Gay-Lussac Method: (Without Indicator Method)

Gay-Lussac method is the method for determining end point in argentometric titration without the use of indicator. It is also referred as **turbidity method**. The end point is marked by cessation of the precipitate formation. The following reaction takes place when sodium bromide (NaBr) solution is titrated with silver nitrate ($AgNO_3$) solution.

$$NaBr + AgNO_3 \longrightarrow AgBr + NaNO_3$$

| Sodium bromide | Silver nitrate | Silver bromide | Sodium nitrate |

It is evident that the precipitation of silver bromide (AgBr) occurs only as long as an excess of Br^- ions is present in solution. Therefore, we can detect accurately the point at which precipitation ceases by taking small portion of the titrated solution at the end of the titrations and adding a single drop of the silver nitrate ($AgNO_3$) solution diluted ten fold.

In this instance detection of end point is made much easier by the fact that near the equivalence point the AgBr precipitate coagulates and collects at the bottom of the vessel in the form of the large curdy flakes. A small quantity of pure barium nitrate may be added to assist the coagulation of precipitate. It is advisable to carry out titration twice, the first titration is used to take appropriate reading. In the second determination silver nitrate ($AgNO_3$) is added drop wise (in about 0.05 ml portion) near the end point to have the exact end point.

Use: The method is commonly used in the estimation of chlorides and bromides as in limit test.

4.13 Titrations Involving Mercuric Nitrate (Hg (NO_3)$_2$)

Method: Fajan's method of precipitation titration.

Indicator used: Sodium nitroprusside Na [Fe (CN)$_5$ NO]

Table 4.3: *Difference between Mohrs and Fajans method*

	Parameters	Mohrs	Fajans method
1.	Indicator used	2% or 5% of K_2CrO_4	Adsorption indicator [0.1% fluorescein, dichlorofluorocein]
2.	Assay performed	NaCl (sodium chloride)	KCl (potassium chloride)
3.	Color change at end point	Yellow-brick red	Yellow → Pink
4.	Solution used for titration	Neutral solution	Acidic or alkaline solution
5.	Process involved	Solubility product	Surface adsorption

Principle: When mercuric nitrate $[Hg(NO_3)_2]$ is added to the solution containing potassium chloride (KCl) along with nitroprusside indicator, a weakly ionized mercuric chloride is formed.

$$Hg\,(NO_3)_2 + 2\,KCl \longrightarrow HgCl_2 + 2\,KNO_3$$

or
$$Hg^{2+} + 2Cl^- \longrightarrow HgCl_2$$

Soluble (weakly ionized)

When all the chloride (Cl^-) ions have been consumed in the solution, further addition of Hg $(NO_3)_2$ makes it to react with sodium nitroprusside to give a white precipitate, indicating the end point.

$$Hg^{+2} + Na_2\,[Fe\,(CN)_5\,NO] \longrightarrow Hg\,[Fe(CN)_5\,NO]^-$$

Sodium nitroprusside $\qquad + 2\,Na^+$

Mercuric nitroprusside (white)

From the reaction;

$$2\,KCl = Hg\,(NO_3)_2 \qquad (MW = 324.63)$$

∴ 2000 ml of 1 M KCl = 324.63 g of Hg $(NO_3)_2$

∴ 1000 ml of 1 M KCl = 162.315 g of Hg $(NO_3)_2$

∴ 1 ml of 1 M KCl $\quad$ = 0.162 g of Hg $(NO_3)_2$

4.14 Titration Involving Thiocyanates: (CNS⁻)

Method: Volhard's method of precipitation titration.

Indicator used: Ferric ammonium sulphate indicator [ferric salt]

Principle: The standard solution of potassium thiocyanate (KCNS) or ammonium thiocyanate (NH_4CNS) in a burette is run into the flask containing solution of silver nitrate ($AgNO_3$) and indicator as ferric NH_4^+ sulphate.

First of all white precipitate of silver thiocyanate (AgCNS) is formed as:

$$Ag^+ + CNS^- \longrightarrow AgCNS\downarrow$$

Silver thiocyanate (white precipitate)

When all the Ag^+ ions present in the solution are completely precipitated, further addition of even a single drop of thiocyanate solution reacts with the Fe^{3+} to give red colored ferric thiocyanate [$Fe(CNS)_3$] marking the end point.

$$Fe^{3+} + 3\,CNS^- \longrightarrow Fe(CNS)_3$$

(Red)

4.15 Assays Involved in Precipitation Titration

1. Direct titration method: The substance in solution is directly titrated with a titrant (precipitant) and completion of precipitation is detected by the use of an internal indicator.

Assay of Sodium Chloride (NaCl)

I.P limit: It contains not less than 99.5% and not more than the equivalent of 100.5% of sodium chloride calculated with reference to the dried substance.

Theory: This method is also called Mohr's method and is applicable if the solution to be titrated is neutral. In acid solution potassium chromate cannot be used as the indicator due to solubility of silver chromate in acids. Sodium chloride is precipitated as silver chloride by adding silver nitrate solution.

$$NaCl + AgNO_3 \longrightarrow AgCl\downarrow + NaNO_3$$

Silver nitrate   Silver chloride
(white precipitate)

When the precipitate formation is completed, a drop of silver nitrate reacts with the indicator, potassium chromate, to form a red precipitate of silver chromate.

$$2\,AgNo_3 + K_2CrO_4 \longrightarrow Ag_2CrO_4 + 2\,KNO_3$$
Silver chromate

Procedure: Accurately weigh sodium chloride (about 0.25 g), is dissolved in water (50 ml) and titrated with 0.1 N silver nitrate ($AgNO_3$) using potassium chromate as an indicator.

Factor: 1 ml of 0.1 N $AgNO_3$ is equivalent to 0.005854 g of NaCl.

2. Residual Titration Method: [Volhard's Method]

In this method excess of standard silver nitrate is added to a solution of halide acidified with nitric acid. The unreacted silver nitrate is titrated with standard ammonium thiocyanate solution using ferric ammonium sulphate as an indicator. At the end point, a permanent red color is developed due to formation of ferric thiocyanate complex.

Assay of Sodium Chloride

Theory: Sodium chloride is precipitated as silver chloride by addition of excess of silver nitrate solution. The precipitate of silver chloride is coagulated by nitrobenzene.

$$NaCl + AgNO_3 \longrightarrow AgCl\downarrow + NaNO_3$$
Silver nitrate   Sodium nitrate

The excess of silver nitrate reacts with ammonium thiocyanate on titration, when whole amount is consumed; a drop of ammonium thiocyanate reacts with ferric ammonium sulphate indicator to give reddish yellow color.

$$AgNO_3 + NH_4SCN \longrightarrow AgSCN + NH_4NO_3$$
Silver nitrate   Silver thiocyanate

$$NH_4SCN + FeNH_4(SO_4)_2 \longrightarrow Fe(SCN)_3 + 2\,(NH_4)_2\,SO_4$$
Ferric thiocyanate (red color)

Procedure: Weigh accurately sodium chloride (0.2 g), dissolve in distilled water (50 ml), and then add 0.1 N silver nitrate solution

(50 ml), nitric acid (3 ml) and nitrobenzene (5 ml). Shake the solution, add ferric ammonium sulphate indicator and titrate with 0.1 N ammonium thiocyanate solution till the color becomes red.
Factor: Each ml of 0.1 N AgNO₃ is equivalent to 0.005845 g of NaCl.

Assay of Ammonium Chloride

I.P limit: It contains not less than 99.5% and not more than the equivalent of 100.5% of NH₄Cl.

Theory: Ammonium chloride (NH₄Cl) is precipitated by adding excess of silver nitrate. The unreacted silver nitrate is estimated by titration with standard ammonium thiocyanate solution. At the end point a drop of ammonium thiocyanate (NH₄SCN) reacts with ferric ammonium sulphate indicator to give red color.

$$NH_4Cl + AgNO_3 \longrightarrow AgCl\downarrow + NH_4NO_3$$

$$\underset{\substack{\text{Ferric ammonium}\\ \text{sulphate}}}{FeNH_4 (SO_4)_2} + NH_4SCN \longrightarrow \underset{\substack{\text{Ferric thiocyanate}\\ \text{(red color)}}}{Fe (SCN)_3} + 2 (NH_4)_2 SO_4$$

Procedure: Accurately weigh ammonium chloride (0.2g), dissolve in distilled water (40 ml), add nitric acid (3 ml), nitrobenzene (5 ml) and 0.1 N silver nitrate (AgNO₃) (50 ml), shake vigorously for 1 minute and titrate with 0.1 N ammonium thiocyanate using ferric ammonium sulphate as the indicator.

Factor: Each ml of 0.1 N AgNO₃ is equivalent to 0.005349 g of NH₄Cl.

EXERCISES

1. What do you understand by precipitation titration?
2. What are the basic conditions necessary for precipitation titration?
3. How many types of precipitation titration are there? Explain in details.
4. Write the titration involving ammonium thiocyanate (NH₄SCN) or potassium thiocyanate (KCNS) and mercuric nitrate (HgNO₃).

5. Define and write the theory of adsorption indicators.
6. What is Volhard's method? Write its applications.
7. Describe Gay Lussac method of determination of end point in precipitation titration.
8. What is solubility product? How does it relate with precipitation titration?
9. Differentiate between Mohr's method and Fajan's method in precipitation titration.
10. Write a note on indicators used in precipitation titrations.
11. Discuss the methods for estimating end point in argentometric titrations.
12. Write preparation and standardization of 0.1 N silver nitrate $(AgNO_3)$.
13. Describe characteristics of a good adsorption indicator.
14. How is the equivalent weight of a precipitant related to its valency?
15. Why is Mohr's method not applicable to the determination of iodates and thiocyantes?
16. Give the factors affecting the solubility of precipitates.

Precipitation Titration, 135

55. Define and write the theory of adsorption indicators.
6. What is Volhard's method? Write its applications.
7. Describe Gay Lussac method of determination of end point

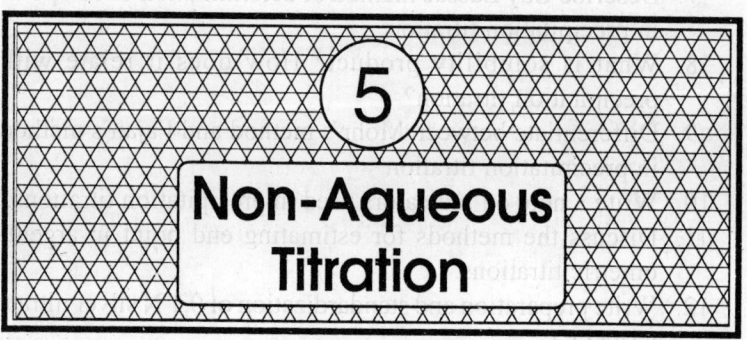

13. Describe characteristics of a good adsorption indicator.
14. How is the equivalent weight of a precipitant related to its

Non-aqueous titration is the titration of substances dissolved in nonaqueous solvents. It is most common titrimetric procedure used in pharmacopoeial assays. The most commonly used procedure is the titration of organic bases with perchloric acid in anhydrous acetic acid. These assays sometimes take some perfecting in terms of being able to judge the end point precisely.

Advantages of Non-Aqueous Titration

1. It is simple and accurate.
2. It is suitable for the titration of very weak acids and bases (acetate and amines).
3. It is a selective titration by using suitable solvent and titrant of acidic/basic component of the physiologically active moiety of the salt.
4. Maintenance of speed, precision, accuracy as par with classical methods of analysis.
5. It enhances the weak reactivity of the substances.
6. It provides a solvent in which organic compounds are soluble.
7. It is possible to titrate mixtures of two or three components selectively with a single titrations by wisdom of right choice of solvent for the non aqueous titrations.
8. Organic acids which are of comparable strength cannot be titrated to each other in aqueous solution but can be titrated

easily in non aqueous solutions. Organic bases follow the same rule.

9. By the proper choice of the solvent or titrant and indicator, "biological ingredients" of a substance whether acidic or basic can be selectively titrated.

The Drugs Which are Assayed by Non Aqueous Titrations Include

- Ephedrine preparations
- Antihistaminics
- Piperazine preparations,
- Preparations containing primary, secondary and tertiary amines (e.g., methyldopa and adrenaline acid tartarate) and
- Preparations containing halogen acid salts (e.g., ephedrine hydrochloride, and chlorpromazine HCl).

5.1 Theory of Non-Aqueous Titration: (Acid-Base Reactions)

The theory is based on fact that water behaves as both a weak acid and a weak base; thus, in an aqueous environment, it can compete effectively with very weak acids and bases with regard to proton donation and acceptance, as shown below:

$$H_2O + H^+ \rightleftharpoons H_3O^+$$
$$\text{(Acid)}$$

Compete with $RNH_2 + H^+ \longrightarrow RNH_3^+$

or $H_2O + B \rightleftharpoons OH^- + BH^+$
$$\text{(Base)}$$

Compete with $ROH + B \longrightarrow RO^- + BH^+$

The reactions which occur during non-aqueous titrations can be explained by means of the concepts of Bronsted-Lowry theory. The theory was formulated independently by its two proponents Johannes Nicolaus Bronsted and Martin Lowry in 1923. It is based upon the idea of protonation of bases through the de-protonation of acids, more commonly referred to as the ability of acids to donate hydrogen ions (H^+) or protons to bases, which accept them.

According to Bronsted and Lowry concept, 'an acid is a substance that tends to lose protons or an acid is a proton donor while a base is a substance that tends to gain proton or a base is a proton acceptor'. According to this definition acids and bases are related as:

$$A \longrightarrow H^+ + B$$

Acid   (Proton)   Base

The acid A, and base B are said to form a 'conjugate pair'.

Conjugate pairs: A pair of substance which can be formed from one another by the gain or lose of proton are called as conjugate pairs. If the pairing is between acid and base, it is known as acid-base conjugate pairs. Every acid has its conjugate base and every base has its conjugate acid. In a given acid-base conjugate pair; at least one member is an ion, e.g.,

(i) $HCl \rightleftharpoons H^+ + Cl^-$

     (Acid)   (Proton)   (Conjugate base)

(ii) $NH_4^+ \rightleftharpoons NH_3 + H^+$

     (Acid)   (Conjugate base)   (Proton)

(iii) $H_3PO_4 \rightleftharpoons H^+ + H_2PO_4^-$

    (Phosphoric   (Proton)   (Conjugate base)
    acid)

(iv) $CH_3 COOH$ (Acid)

$$H^+ + CH_3COO^-$$

Proton   Conjugate Base

A conjugate base could be electrically neutral, e.g., ammonia (NH_3).

(a) $NH_3 + H^+ \rightleftharpoons NH_4^+$

(b) $SO_4^{2-} + H^+ \rightleftharpoons H SO_4^- + H^+ \rightleftharpoons H_2SO_4$ [Acid]

(c) $H_2PO_4^- + H^+ \rightleftharpoons H_3PO_4$

(Base)   (Proton)   (Conjugate base)

To express the relationship between conjugate acid/base pairs, the following relationship is used:

$$Acid_1 + Base_2 \rightleftharpoons Acid_2 + Base_1$$

Where $Base_1$: Conjugate base of $Acid_1$.

$Acid_2$: Conjugate acid of $Base_2$.

For example;

$$Acid_1 + Base_2 \rightleftharpoons Acid_2 + Base_1$$

$$HCl + H_2O \rightleftharpoons H_3O^+ + Cl^-$$

$$H_3PO_4 + H_2O \rightleftharpoons H_3O^+ + H_2PO_4^-$$

$$NH_4^+ + H_2O \rightleftharpoons H_3O^+ + NH_3$$

$$HNO_3 + NH_3 \rightleftharpoons NH_4^+ + NO_3^-$$

Since the acids HNO_3, HCl and HBr are stronger acids than H_3O^+, thus forward reaction are almost complete, according to the Bronstered Lowry concept. Thus, we see in water, the acids like HNO_3, HCl and HBr show equal strength. This is due to the fact that H_2O acts as a base, strong enough to dissociate the above acids to the completion. Hence, water is called levelling agent because it levels them to the same strength and the phenomenon is called **levelling effect of H_2O.**

However, if we take the weaker base than water like CH_3COOH, the dissociation of all the acids will not be completed to such extent. Hence, the dissociation of all the acids will not be completed to the same extent, and the strength of the acids will be differentiated. Thus, CH_3COOH acts as differentiating agent and the phenomenon is called **differentiating effect of CH_3COOH.**

Table 5.1: *Some common conjugate acids and bases in order of their relative strength*

	Conjugate acids	Conjugate bases	
Strongest			Weakest
	$HClO_4$	ClO_4^-	
	H_2SO_4	HSO_4^-	
	HCl	Cl^-	
Strength increasing	H_3O^+	H_2O	Strength increasing
	HSO_4^-	SO_4^{2-}	
	HF	F^-	
	CH_3COOH	CH_3COO^-	
	H_2S	HS^-	
	NH_4^+	NH_3	
	HCO_3^-	CO_3^{2-}	
	H_2O	OH^-	
	HS^-	S^{2-}	
	OH^-	O^{2-}	
Weakest			Strongest

Molecules or ions that can behave both as Bronsted acids and bases are called amphiprotic substances. Examples are water (H_2O) and bicarbonate (HCO^-_3).

With HCl, water acts as a base in accepting a proton from the acid,

$$HCl + H_2O \rightleftharpoons H_3O^+ + Cl^-$$

However, water is an acid donating a proton to ammonia (NH_3)

$$\underset{(Base)}{NH_3} + H_2O \rightleftharpoons \underset{(Acid)}{NH_4^+ + OH^-}$$

The strongest acid has higher tendency to denote proton and will always produce weak conjugate base and weak acid will produce strong conjugate base and vice versa.

$$\underset{(Strong\ acid)}{HCl} + H_2O \rightleftharpoons H_3O^+ + \underset{(Weak\ conjugate\ base)}{Cl^-}$$

$$CH_3COOH + H_2O \rightleftharpoons H_3O^+ + CH_3COO^-$$

(Weak acid)   (Base)   (Acid)   (Strong conjugate base)

Same case is with strong and weak bases as:

$$NH_3 + H_2O \rightleftharpoons NH_4^+ + OH^-$$

(Weak conjugate acid)

HCO^-_3 can act as both Bronsted acid and base because it can donate a proton to form CO_3^{-2} and it can accept the proton to form H_2CO_3.

5.2 Solvents in Non-Aqueous Titration

Various organic solvents may be used to replace water to they compete less effectively with the analyte for proton donation or acceptance. They are:

1. Aprotic solvents: These are chemically inert organic solvents like benzene and chloroform. They have a low dielectric constant and do not ionize other compounds. Picric acid forms a colorless solution in benzene which becomes yellow on adding aniline since the acid does not dissociate in benzene solution and in the presence of the base aniline, it acts as an acid.

2. Protophobic solvent: These are basic in character and form solvated protons on reaction with acids.

$$HB + \text{basic solvent} \longrightarrow \text{Solvated proton} + B^-$$

A weakly basic solvent has fewer tendencies to accept a proton than a strongly basic one. Similarly, a weak acid has less tendency to donate protons than a strong acid such as perchloric acid exhibits more strongly acidic properties than a weak acid such as acetic acid when dissolved in a weakly basic solvent. All acids tend to become typical in strength when dissolve in strongly basic solvents due to the greater affinity of strong bases for protons. Strong bases are levelling solvents for acids; weak bases are differentiating solvents for acids.

3. Protophilic solvents: These solvents are basic in character and had a strong tendency to bind with proton of an acid to form solvated proton.

$$HCl + NH_3 \rightleftharpoons [NH_4^+] + [Cl^-]$$

Solvated proton

4. Amphiprotic solvents: These solvents have both protophilic and protogenic properties. Examples are water, acetic acid and the alcohols. They are dissociated to a slight extent. The dissociation of acetic acid, which is frequently used as a solvent for titration of basic substances, is shown in the equation below:

$$CH_3COOH \rightleftharpoons CH_3COO^- + H^+$$

Here the acetic acid is functioning as an acid. If a very strong acid such as perchloric acid is dissolved in acetic acid, the latter can function as a base and combine with protons donated by the perchloric acid to form an 'onium' ion.

$$HClO_4 \rightleftharpoons [ClO_4^-] + [H^+]$$

$$CH_3COOH + H^+ \rightleftharpoons CH_3COOH_2^+ \text{ (Onium ion)}$$

Since the onium ion readily donated its proton to a base, a solution of perchloric acid in glacial acetic acid functions as a strongly acidic solution. When a weak base, such as pyridine, is dissolved in acetic acid, the acetic acid exerts its levelling effect and enhances the basic properties of the pyridine. It is possible, therefore, to titrate a solution of a weak base in acetic acid with perchloric acid ($HClO_4$), and obtain a sharp end point when attempts to carry out the titration in aqueous solution are unsuccessful. The various reactions with perchloric acid, acetic acid and pyridine are summarized below:

$$CH_3COOH + HClO_4 \rightleftharpoons CH_3COOH_2^+ + ClO_4^-$$

$$CH_3COOH + C_6H_5N \rightleftharpoons CH_3COO^- + C_6H_5NH^+$$

$$CH_3COOH_2^+ + CH_3COO^- \rightleftharpoons 2\,CH_3COOH$$

Sum up: $HClO_4 + C_6H_5N \rightleftharpoons C_6H_5NH^+ + ClO_4^-$

5.3 Methodology

For non-aqueous titration, the following four steps are usually taken into consideration:

Step 1: Preparation of 0.1 N perchloric acid: Perchloric acid (72%, 8.5 ml) is slowly added with shaking to glacial acetic acid (900 ml). Then acetic anhydride (30 ml) is added and the volume adjusted to 1 litre with glacial acetic acid. The solution is allowed to stand for 24 hours before use. The acetic anhydride reacts with water present with perchloric acid and acetic acid to give an anhydrous solution. The perchloric acid must be well diluted with acetic acid before adding acetic anhydride, otherwise explosive acetyl perchlorate may be formed.

Precautions: The following precautions must be observed:

1. Conversion of acetic anhydride into acetic acid requires 40–45 minutes for its completion. It being a exothermic reaction, the solution must be allowed to cool at room temperature before adding the glacial acetic acid solution.
2. Perchloric acid is not only a powerful oxidizing agent but also a strong acid. Hence, it must be handled very carefully.
3. Avoid adding an excess of acetic anhydride especially when primary and secondary amines are to be assayed because they may rapidly convert into their corresponding acetylated non-basic products.

Step 2: Standardization of 0.1 N perchloric acid: Alkali and alkaline earth metal salts of organic acid act as bases in acetic acid solution.

$$R\,COOM \rightleftharpoons RCOO^- + M^+$$

$$CH_3COOH_2^+ + RCOO^- \rightleftharpoons RCOOH + CH_3COOH$$

In usual practices, potassium hydrogen phthalate may be used as a standardizing agent for acetous perchloric acid.

Potassium hydrogen phthalate   Phthalic acid

Therefore, 204.14 g of $C_8H_5O_4K \equiv HClO_4 \equiv 1000$ mlN

or, 0.02041 g of $C_8H_5O_4K \equiv 1$ ml 0.1 N $HClO_4$

Procedure: Accurately weighed quantity of potassium hydrogen phthalate (0.5 g) is poured into a 100 ml conical flask. A reflux condenser is attached with silica gel drying tube. Glacial acetic acid (25 ml) is added warmed to dissolve salt, cooled and titrated with 0.1 N perchloric acid using 2 drops of an indicator such as 0.5% acetous crystal violet (end point blue to green) or 0.5% acetous oracet blue B (end point blue to pink) or a-naphthobenzein [0.2 % in glacial acetic acid (end point blue to dark green)] or quinaldine red [(0.1% in methanol) (end point magenta to almost colourless)]. The same indicator must be used throughout for standardization. The end point may be determined by titrating potentiometrically.

Step 3: Effect of temperature: A small temperature variation can resulted in significant errors unless suitable correction factors are used. Therefore, standardization and titration should be carried out at the same temperature. If there is a temperature difference, the volume of titrant may be corrected by applying the following formula:

$$V_a = V_b [1 + 0.001 (t_1 - t_2)]$$

where, V_a = corrected volume of titrant,

V_b = volume of titrant measured,

t_1 = temperature of which titrant was standardized, and

t_2 = temperature at which titration was carried.

Table 5.2: Indicators used in non-aqueous titrations

S. No.	Indicator	Color change basic	Color change neutral	Color change acidic
1	Crystal violet (0.5 percent in glacial acetic acid)	violet	blue-green	yellowish-green
2	α-Naptholbenzein (0.2 per cent in glacial acetic acid)	blue or blue-green	orange	dark-green
3	Oracet Blue B (0.5 percent in glacial acetic acid)	blue	purple	pink
4	Quinaldine red (0.1 percent in methanol)	mage-nta	....	almost colorless

Step 4: Choice of Indicators in Non-Aqueous: A number of indicators stated in Table 5.2 are commonly used in non-aqueous titrations. It is, however, necessary to mention here that the same indicators must be used throughout for carrying out the standardization, titration and neutralization of mercuric acetate solution.

5.4 Assay By Non -Aqueous Titration

Assay of various pharmaceutical substances either in pure form or in dosage form to be assayed are carried out successfully by non aqueous titrations. For the sake of convenience these typical titrations can be categorized into two broad groups, namely:

1. Acidimetry in non-aqueous titration: (Titration of amines and halogen acid salts).

2. Alkalimetry in non-aqueous titration: (Titration of acidic substances).

1. Acidimetry in Non Aqueous Titration

(Titration of amines and halogen acid salts).

(i) Amines

(a) Methyldopa: In general, the reaction taking place between a primary amine and perchloric acid may be expressed as follows:

$$R.NH_2 \ + \ HClO_4 \ \longrightarrow \ [R.NH_3]^+ + ClO_4^-$$

Amine   Perchloric acid

The specific reaction between methyldopa and perchloric acid is expressed by the following equations:

Hence, 211.24 g of $C_{10}H_{13}NO_4 \equiv HClO_4 \equiv H \equiv 1000$ ml N

0.12112 g of $C_{10}H_{13}NO_4 \equiv 1$ ml of $HClO_4$

Procedure: Weigh accurately about 0.2 g of methyldopa and dissolve in 15 ml of anhydrous formic acid, 30 ml of glacial acetic acid and 30 ml of dioxane. Add 0.1 ml of crystal violet solution and titrate with 0.1 N perchloric acid. Perform a blank determination and make any necessary corrections.

Equivalent factor: Each 1 ml of 0.1 N perchloric acid is equivalent to 0.02112 g of $C_{10}H_{13}NO_4$

Reaction involved:

Methyldopa   Perchloric acid

Calculations: The percentage of the methyldopa present in a sample is given by:

$$\% \text{ methyldopa} = \frac{ml \times 0.1 \times 0.01221 \times 100}{\text{Weight of sample}}$$

The estimation of weak base can be performed in glacial acetic acid using perchloric acid as the titrant. End point is detected by using an indicator or by potentiometric method.

(b) Adrenaline acid tartarate: In general, the reaction taking place between a primary amine and perchloric acid may be expressed as follows:

$$R.NH_2 + HClO_4 \longrightarrow [R.NH_3]^+ + ClO_4^-$$

Hence, 183.2 g of $C_{19}H_{13}NO_3 \equiv HClO_4 \equiv H \equiv 1000$ ml N

0.01832 g of $C_{19}H_{13}NO_3 \equiv$ ml of $HClO_4$

Procedure: Weigh accurately about 0.3 g of adrenaline acid tartarate and dissolve in 15 ml of anhydrous formic acid, 30 ml of glacial acetic acid and 30 ml of dioxane. Add 0.1 ml of crystal violet solution and titrate with 0.1 N perchloric acid. Perform a blank determination and make any necessary corrections.

Equivalent factor: Each ml of 0.1N perchloric acid is equivalent to 0.02112 g of $C_{19}H_{13}NO_3$

Calculations: The percentage of adrenaline acid tartarate present in a sample is given by:

$$\% \text{ adrenaline acid tartarate } = \frac{ml \times 0.1 \times 0.01221 \times 100}{\text{Weight of sample}}$$

The estimation of weak base can be performed in glacial acetic acid using perchloric acid as the titrant. End point is detected by using an indicator or by potentiometric method.

(ii) Titration of Halogen Acid Salts of Bases

In general the halide ions are very weakly basic in character and they cannot react quantitatively with aqueous perchloric acid. In order to overcome this problem mercuric acetate is usually added to a halide salt thereby causing the replacement of halide ion by an equivalent amount of acetate ion, which serves as a strong base in acetic acid as shown below:

$$2\,RHN_2.HCl \rightleftharpoons 2\,RHN_3{}^+ + 2Cl^-$$
$$(CH_3COO)_2\,Hg \text{ (undissociated)} + 2Cl^- \rightarrow HgCl_2 + 2CH_3COO^-$$
$$2CH_3COO^- + 2CH_3COOH \rightarrow 4CH_3COOH$$

Assay of Ephedrine Hydrochloride Tablets

Theory: Ephedrine hydrochloride is too weakly basic to react quantitatively with acetous perchloric acid. Addition of mercuric acetate to halide salt replaces ion by an equivalent quantity of acetate ion which is a strong base in acetic acid and can react quantitatively with perchloric acid.

$$2\,C_{10}H_{15}NO.HCl \rightleftharpoons 2\,C_{10}H_{16}N^+O.2Cl^-$$
Ephedrine hydrochloride

$$(CH_3COO)_2\,Hg \text{ (undissociated)} + 2Cl^- \rightarrow HgCl_2 + 2CH_3COO^-$$
$$2CH_3COO^- + 2CH_3COOH \rightarrow 4CH_3COOH$$

Factor: Each 1 ml of perchloric acid is equivalent to 0.0217 g of $C_{10}H_{15}NO.HCl$

Procedure: Weigh accurately 20 tablets and grind to fine powder. A quantity of powder equivalent to about 0.15 g of ephedrine hydrochloride is mixed with glacial acetic acid (30 ml), mercuric acetate solution (10 ml) and crystal-violet solution (0.1ml). Warm gently the solution, cool and titrate with 0.1 N perchloric acid until the violet color changes to green blue. Perform the blank titration in the same way.

2. Alkalimetry in Non-Aqueous Titration (Titration of Acidic Substances)

A plethora of weakly acidic pharmaceutical substances may be effectively titrated by making use of a suitable non-aqueous solvent with the sharp end point. The wide spectrum of such organic compounds include: anhydrides, acids, amino acids, acid halides, enols, xanthines, sulphonamides, phenols, imides and organic salts of the inorganic acids. However, a weak inorganic acid can be estimated conveniently employing ethylenediamine as the non-aqueous solvent.

Preparation of 0.1 M Sodium Methoxide Solution

Cool down anhydrous methanol (150 ml) in ice- cold water and add freshly cut sodium metal (about 2.5 g) in portions. When the metal has dissolved, add sufficient amount toluene, previously dried over sodium wire, to produce 1000 ml.

Standardization of 0.1 M Sodium Methoxide Solution with Benzoic Acid

Standardize the solution in the following manner immediately before use. Dissolve accurately weighted benzoic acid (0.4 g) in dimethyl formamide (80 ml), add thymolphthalein solution (0.15 ml) and titrate with 0.1 M sodium methoxide solution to a blue end point.

A blank titration is also performed on the solvent system to account for acidic impurity in dimethyl formamide and the correction is made accordingly.

Factor: Each ml of 0.1 M sodium methoxide is equivalent to 0.01221 g of benzoic acid.

EXERCISES

1. What are non-aqueous titrations? Give some important advantages.
2. What do you understand by levelling and differentiating effects?
3. Discuss briefly about Bronsted and Lowry concept of non-aqueous titrations.
4. Write the preparation and standardization of 0.1 N perchloric acid ($HClO_4$).
5. Describe the preparation and standardization of 0.1 N sodium methoxide solution.
6. Give a note on solvents used in non-aqueous titrations.
7. Explain the assay procedure of
    (i) Ephedrine HCl
    (ii) Methyldopa
    (iii) Adrenaline acid tartarate.
8. Mention some indicators used in non-aqueous titrations.
9. Discuss the effect of temperature on assays in non aqueous titrations.
10. Write a note on
    (i) Acidimetry in non-aqueous titrations.
    (ii) Alkalimetry in non-aqueous titrations.

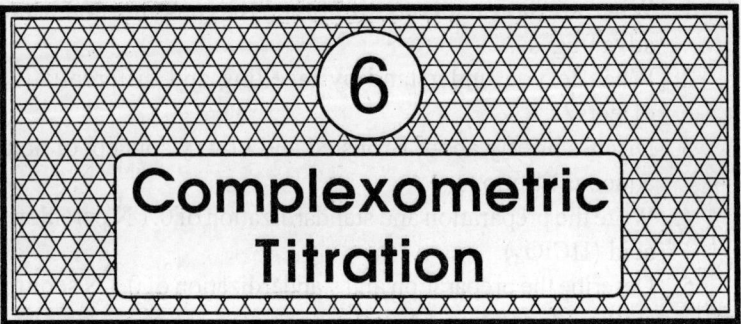

6
Complexometric Titration

Complexometric titration is a type of titration based on reaction between a ligand and a matel ion to form a complex. Complexometric titrations are particularly useful for determination of a mixture of different metal ions in solution. An indicator with a marked color change is usually used to detect the end-point of the titration. Any complexation reaction can theortically be applied as a volumetric technique provided that:

1. The reaction reaches equilibrium rapidly following each addition of titrant.

2. Interfering situations do not arise (such as stepwise formation of various complexes resulting in the presence of more than one complex in solution in significant concentration during the titration process).

3. A complexometric indicator capable of locating equivalence point with fair accuracy is available.

The formation of complex during a chemical reaction may serve as the basis of titrimetric assay. A complexation reaction with a metal ion involves the replacement of one or more of the coordinated solvent molecules by other nucleophilic groups. A complexing agent is any electron-donating ion or molecule, called **ligand**, which produces one or more covalent bonds with the metal and forms a complex which has different properties from those of the free metal ions. Complex formation takes place in the titration of a solution of cyanide with silver nitrate or of chloride ion with mercury (II) nitrate solution.

$$2\,CN^- + Ag^+ \rightleftharpoons [Ag(CN)_2]$$

$$2\,CN^- + Hg^{2+} \rightleftharpoons [Hg(CN)_2]$$

Ligand anion   Metal cation   Stable complex ion

The complexing agent holds a metal ion in complex through one or more co-ordinate or covalent bonds. There are a specific number of ligands that are bound to each metal ion. This is based on a specific co-ordination number, which varies for each metal ion. A metal ion has more than one co-ordination number. The ferricyanide ion may be consisted of three ordinary covalent and three co-ordinate bonds. In a complex the bonds are identical hybrid bonds which are directed towards the apices of a regular octahedron.

Complexes involving simple ligands forming only one bond are called **co-ordination compounds.** Ligands having two or more electron-donating groups are known as **chelating agents** forming cyclic structures. 1,2-Diaminoethane behave like two ammonia molecules and forms chelates with copper and cobalt ions. Organic compounds containing groups with an easily replaceable proton (–COOH, phenolic OH) form chelates. The greater the number of rings, which can be formed, the more stable will be the chelates. The solubility of metal chelates in water depends upon the presence of hydrophilic groups such as –COOH, –SO_3H, –NH_2 and –OH. When both acidic and basic groups are present, complex will be soluble over a wide range of pH. Ethylenediamine tetra acetic acid (EDTA) is a very important reagent for complex formation titration. Dimethylglyoxime and salicylaldoxime form water-insoluble complexes, which are soluble inorganic solvents. Complexes of most divalent metals are stable in ammonia solution. Trivalent metal complexes are still more firmly bound and stable in strongly acidic solutions. For example, the cobalt (Co^{3+}) edetate complex is stable in concentrated hydrochloric acid. Increase in temperature causes a slight increase in the ionization of the complex and a slight lowering of stability constant.

Color of complexes: There is a change in the absorption spectrum when complexes are formed which is a basis of many colorimetric assays.

6.1 Complexometric Titration with EDTA

Ethylenediamine tetraacetic acid, more commonly known as EDTA, belongs to a class of synthetic compounds known as polyaminocarboxylic acids. Acting as a ligand that shows multiple coordination sites, EDTA forms very strong 1:1 stiochoimetric complexes with metal ions of valency +2 and other higher charged metal ions in aqueous solution. EDTA (ethylene diamine tetra acetic acid) has four carboxyl groups and two amine groups that can act as electron pair donors, or Lewis bases (Fig. 6.1). The ability of EDTA is to donate its six lone pairs of electrons for the formation of coordinate covalent bonds to metal cations and makes EDTA a hexadentate ligand. However, in practice EDTA is usually only partially ionized, and thus forms fewer than six coordinate covalent bonds with metal cations. Disodium EDTA, commonly used in the standardization of aqueous solutions of transition metal cations, only forms four coordinate covalent bonds to metal cations at pH values less than or equal to 12. In this range of pH values the amine groups remain protonated and thus unable to donate electrons to the formation of coordinate covalent bonds. In analytical chemistry the shorthand "Na_2H_2Y" is typically used to designate disodium EDTA. This shorthand can be used to designate any species of EDTA. The "Y" stands for the EDTA molecule, and the "H_n" designates the number of acidic protons bonded to the EDTA molecule. EDTA forms an octahedral complex with most 2^+ metal cations, M^{2+}, in aqueous solution. The main reason that EDTA is used so extensively in the standardization of metal cation solutions is that the formation constant for most metal cation-EDTA complexes is very high and the equilibrium for the reaction lies far to the right.

$$M^{2+} + H_4Y \longrightarrow MH_2Y + 2H^+$$

Carrying out the reaction in a basic buffer solution removes H^+ as it is formed, which also drives the reaction to the right. For most purposes it can be considered that the formation of the metal cation-EDTA complex goes to completion, and this is chiefly why EDTA is used in titrations and standardizations of most solutions of transistion metal ions.

6.2 Titration of Metal Ions Using Disodium Edetate

Disodium edetate acid is sparingly soluble in water. During titration the diedetate solution is run into a solution of a metal ion buffered to promote efficient complex formation. The end point of complexo- metric titrations is shown by means of **pM indicator** (negative log of metal ion concentration) which is a dye capable of acting as a chelating agent to give a dye-metal complex. The dye-metal complex is different in color and forms the dye itself. When there is the slightest excess of edentate, the metal-dye complex decomposes to produce free dye, this is accomplished by a change in color. In complexometric titrations, a metal-ion indicator shows the color due to the dye-metal complex until the end point when an equivalent amount of EDTA titrant has been added. When there is a slight excess of EDTA titrant,the dye-metal complex decomposes to form free dye and there is a change in color, which is dependent on pH of the solution. The pH variation also affects the stability of the complex. Therefore, a buffer solution is used to maintain the required pH during the titration. To carry out metal cation titrations using disodium EDTA, it is almost always necessary to use a complexometric indicator, usually an organic

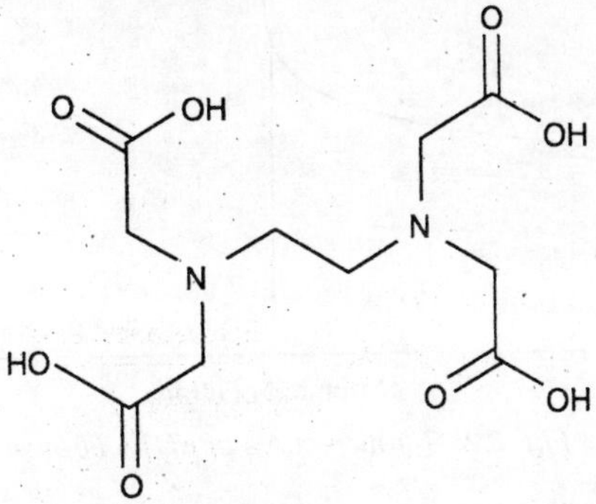

Fig. 6.1: EDTA

dye such as Fast Sulphon Black, Eriochrome Black T, Eriochrome Red B or Murexide, to determine the end point. These dyes bind to the metal cations in solution to form colored complexes. However, since EDTA binds to metal cations much more strongly than does the dye used as an indicator, the EDTA will displace the dye from the metal cations as it is added to the solution of analyte. A color change in the solution being titrated indicates that all of the dye has been displaced from the metal cations in solution, and that the end point has been reached.

6.3 Theory and Titration Curve of Complexometry

Many theories of acid base titrations are used in complexometry. In complexometric titrations the free metal ion disappears as they are changed into complex ion. Any method which can determine this sudden disappearance of free metal ion can be used for detecting the end point in the complexometric titration. End point can be detected visually with an indicator. For complexometry curves we plot $pM= -\log [M^{n+}]$ versus volume of titrant added, we find that at the end point the pM rapidly increases. This sudden pM rise results from the removal of last traces of free metal ions from solution of EDTA. Two parameters are important in determining the magnitude of the break on the titration curve at the end point

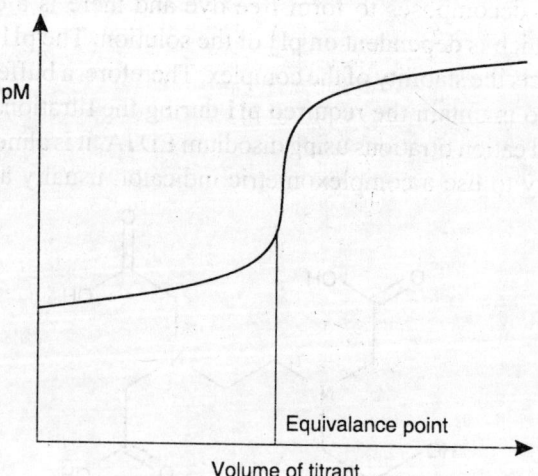

Fig. 6.2: Titration curve of EDTA titration

1. Stability of the complex formed.
2. Number of steps involved in complex formation.

Greater the stability constant for the complex formed, the larger would be the change in the free metal concentration (pM) at the equivalence point and thus more clear would be the end point.

6.4 Effect of pH on Complexometric Titration

During a complexometric titration the pH must be kept constant by the use of buffer solution. Control of pH is important since the H^+ plays an important role in the chelation. Most ligands are bases and bind hydrogen ions throughout a wide pH range. Some of these H^+ are frequently displaced from the ligand by the metal during chelate formation.

$$M^{2+} + H_2 EDTA^{2-} \rightleftharpoons M-EDTA^{2-} + 2H^+$$

Therefore, the stability of the metal complex is pH dependent. Lower the pH of the solution less would be the stability of the complex because more H^+ are available to compete with the metal ion for the ligand. Only metals that form very stable complexes with titrant can be titrated.

6.5 Types of EDTA Complexometric Titration

EDTA titrations have been performed to nearly all common cations. The important types of EDTA titration of metal ion are:

1. **Direct titrations:** The direct titration with EDTA may be performed on many cations using metallochromic indicators. The metal ion in solution is buffered to the desired pH and titrated directly with the standard EDTA solution. Precipitation of the metal hydroxide is prevented by adding some auxilliary complexing agent. At the equivalence point, the concentration of metal ion (being determined) decreases rapidly. This is generally determined by a change in color of metal indicator which responds the change in pM. The total hardness of water is determined by direct titration with EDTA using Eriochrome Black T as indicator.
2. **Back titration:** In such cases an excess of standard EDTA solution is added, the resulting solution is buffered to the

desired pH, and the excess of the reagent is back titrated with a standard metal ion solution, usually a solution of zinc chloride or sulphate is often used. The end point is detected with the aid of metal indicator which responds to the metal ion introduced in back titration. This method is also used to determine metals in precipitates, for example, aluminum, lead (Pb) in $PbSO_4$ and calcium in CaC_2O_4.

3. **Replacement titration:** Such titrations are used for metal ions, which do not react with the metal indicator, or for metal ions which form EDTA complexes that are more stable than those of the other metals such as Mg^{2+} and Ca^{2+}. The metal cation M^{n+} to be determined is treated with Mg-EDTA complex, when the reaction occurs:

$$M^{2+} + MgY^{2-} \longrightarrow MY^{(n-4)} + Mg^{2+}$$

$$M^{2+} + H_2Y^{2-} \longrightarrow M\text{-EDTA}$$

4. **Alkalimetric titrations:** When a solution of disodium salt (EDTA), Na_2H_2Y, is added to a solution of metal ion, complexes are formed and two equivalent of hydrogen ions are set free:

$$M^{2+} + MgY^{2-} \longrightarrow MY^{(n-4)} + Mg^{2+}$$

These liberated hydrogen ions can be titrated with a standard solution of sodium hydroxide (NaOH) using a usual acid-base indicator to locate the end point. It may also be determined by potentiometric titrations. Also, an iodate-iodide mixture may be added along with the EDTA solution and the iodine set free may be titrated with the standard thiosulphate solution.

6.6 Indicators Used in Complexometric Titration (Table 6.1)

A **complexometric indicator** is an ionochromic dye that undergoes a definite color change in the presence of specific metal ions. It forms a weak complex with the ions present in the solution, which has significantly different color than the form existing outside of the complex. In analytical chemistry, complexometric indicators are used in complexometric titration to indicate the exact moment when all the metal ions in the solution are sequestered by a chelating agent (most usually EDTA). Such indicators are also called **metallochromic indicators**. The indicator may be present in another liquid phase in equilibrium with the titrated phase of the indicator and it is described as **extraction indicator**. Some complexometric indicators are sensitive to air and are destroyed. When such solution lose color during titration, a drop or two of fresh indicator may have to be added. Complexometric indicators are water-soluble organic molecules and such metal indicators should comply with the following requirements:

- It should be chemically stable during storage and throughout the titration,
- It should form 1:1 complex which must be weaker than the metal chelate complex,
- It must have sufficient stability to withstand dilution and still give an adequate color change at the end point,
- Color of the indicator and the metal complex should be different to locate the end point,
- Color reaction should be selective for the metal being titrated, and
- It should not compete with the titrant.

Action of Complexometric or Organochromic Indicators

Let the metal be denoted by M, indicator by I and chelate by EDTA. At the start of titration, the reaction medium contains the metal indicator complex (MI) and excess of metal ions. When EDTA titrant is added to the system a competitive reaction takes place between the free metal ion and EDTA. Since the metal indicator complex is weaker than the metal-EDTA chelate, the EDTA which is being added during the course of the titration is chelating the free metal ion in solution at the expense of the MI complex. Finally at the end point, EDTA removes the last traces of the metal from the indicator and the indicator changes from its complexed color to its metal free color. The overall reaction is given by:

$$MI + M + EDTA \longrightarrow M - EDTA + I \text{ (Metal free colour)}$$

Where MI = metal indicator complex, M= metal indicator and I = indicator.

Many compounds have been used as indicators for complexometric titrations. They are:

(1) Alizarin Fluorine Blue

It is used in acid solution at pH 4.3 for the titration of lead (Pb^{2+}), zinc (Zn^{2+}), cobalt (Co^{2+}), mercury (Hg^{2+}) and copper (Cu^{2+}) when

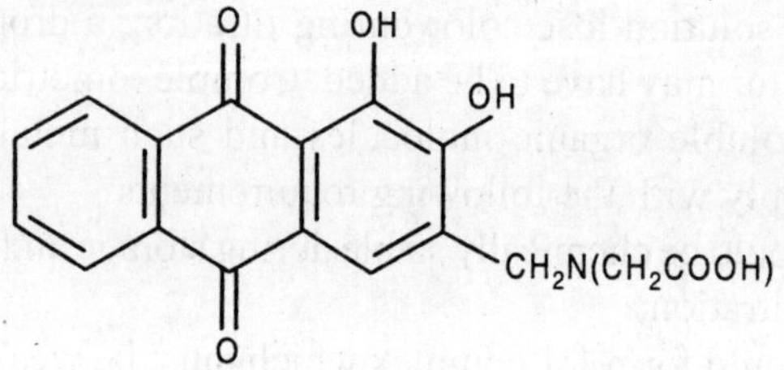

Fig. 6.3: *Alizarin fluorine blue*

the color changes from red to yellow. It is also used in the determination of fluorine in some synthetic drugs (Fig. 6.3).

(2) Sodium Alizarin Sulphonate

It yields a bluish-red color with aluminum, and thorium ions at pH 4.0 and a yellow in the absence of these ions. It is used to determine fluorine in Triamcinolone (synthetic corticosteriod) by titration with standard thorium nitrate solution.

(3) Murexide

Murexide is ammonium purpurate which is used for the titration of calcium at pH 12. Calcium is bound in an eight membered ring in the murexide chelate which is less stable in comparison to five and six membered ring chelates. Since magnesium–murexide in less stable then the calcium complex,

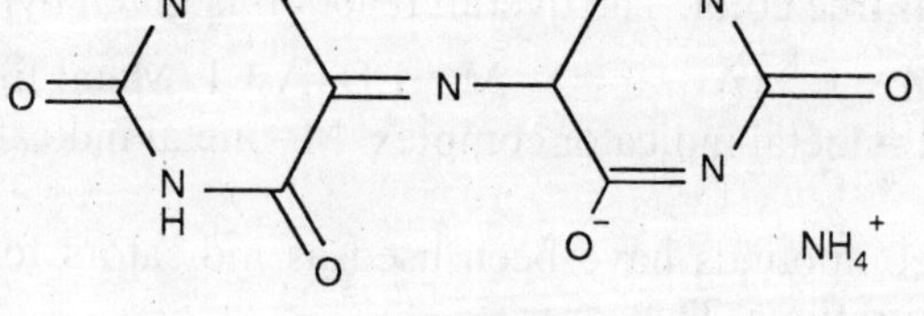

Fig. 6.4: *Murexide*

calcium is titrated in the presence of magnesium as in water analysis. Copper, cobalt and cerium form yellow complexes with murexide in alkaline solution. They give clear color changes when titrated with sodium edetate (Fig. 6.4).

(4) Eriochrome Black T

This indicator is blue at about pH 10 and most of its complexes are red. Below pH 6.3 and above pH 11.5 the dye itself is red. The

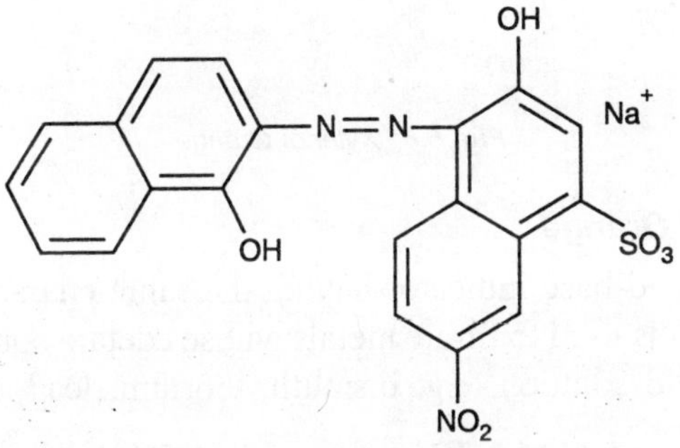

Fig. 6.5: Eriochrome black T

titration is carried out in the presence of a buffer at pH 10. Magnesium, calcium, zinc, manganese, lead and mercury are titrated directly using this indicator. Cobalt nickel, copper, aluminum, silver, titanium and platinum form pre stable complexes with the dye than with the edetate (Fig. 6.5).

(5) Catechol Violet

The catechols form weak, highly-colored complexes in neutral, acid and alkaline solutions. All the complexes are blue in alkaline solution. In this solution, clear end points are shown with magnesium, manganese, iron, nickel, zinc, cadmium and calcium.

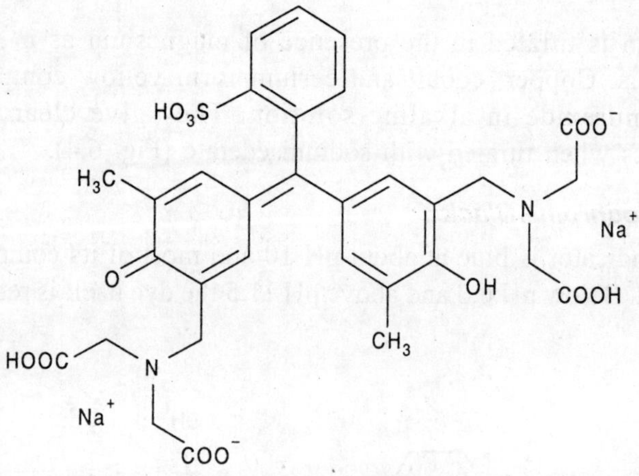

Fig. 6.6: Xylenol Orange

(6) Xylenol Orange

This is an acid-base indicator having the same characteristics as cresol red. It is used to titrate metals whose edetate complexes are stable in acid solution, e.g. bismuth, thorium, lead, lanthanum,

Table 6.1: *Complexometric indicators*

S. No.	Indicator	Color change	pH range	Metal detected
1.	Eriochrome Black T	Red to Blue	6–7	Ca, Ba, Mg,and Pb.
2.	Murexide	Violet to blue	12	Ca, Cu and Co
3.	Catechol-violet	Violet to red	10	Mg, Mn and Co
4.	Methyl thymol blue	Blue to yellow	4–5	Hg, Zn, Pb, and Co
5.	Diphenyl carbazone	Violet colored complex	8–9	Hg, methyluracil
6	Alizarin	Red to yellow	4.3	Co, Ba, Mg, Cu^{2+}, Mn, and Pb.

cadmium and mercury. The stability of the complexes varies with pH (Fig. 6.6).

(7) Calcein

Also known as **fluorexon, fluorescein complex,** is a fluorescent dye with an excitation and emission wavelengths of 495/515nm, respectively. Calcein also self-quenches at concentrations above 100mM. It is used as a complexometric indicator for titration of calcium ions with EDTA, and for fluorometric determination of calcium. It has the appearance of orange crystals (Fig. 6.7).

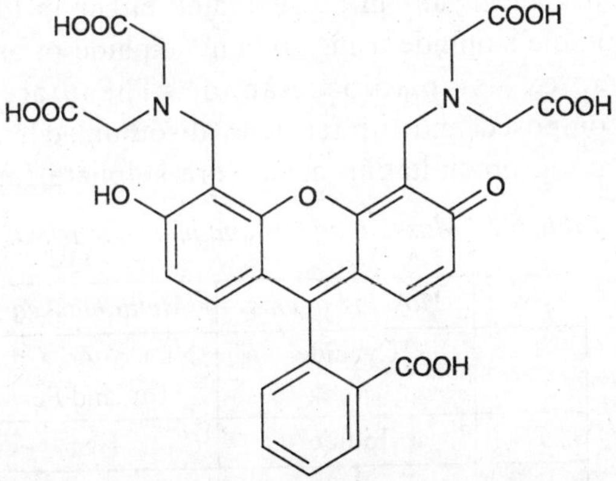

Fig. 6.7: Calcein

(8) Diphenylcarbazone

It is used an indicator for determination of mercury in methylthiouracil. It forms a blue color with ferric iron between pH 2 and 5, a violet color between pH 5.7 and 7 and a red complex in alkaline solution (Fig. 6.8).

$$C_6H_5N = NCONHC_6H_5$$

Fig. 6.8: Diphenycarbazone

(9) Methyl Thymol Blue

It is derived form of thymol blue and used for bismuth in strongly acid solution and for lead, zinc, cadmium, mercury and cobalt in weakly acid solution.

6.7 Masking and Demasking Agents

Owing to the wide range of cations complexed by disodium EDTA, the selectivity of the method is poor and metal impurities may be titrated with the ion. When it is required to assay one or more ion in a mixture of cations and to eliminate the effects of possible impurities, masking agents are used. Masking agents act either by precipitation or by formation of complexes which are more stable than the interfering ion edetate complex (Table 6.2).

1. **Masking by precipitation**: Many heavy metals, e.g., cobalt, copper and lead can be separated either in the form of insoluble sulphide using sodium sulphide or as insoluble complex using thioacetamide. These are filtered, decomposed and titrated with disodium edetate. Other common precipitating agents are sulphate for lead and

Table 6.2: *Masking agents and metals masked.*

S. No.	Masking agents	Metal masked
1.	Cyanide	Ni, Co, Zn, Cd, Cu, and Fe
2.	Iodide	Hg
3.	Ascorbic acid	Fe and Cu
4.	Triethanolamine	Fe, Al, Mn

barium, oxalate for calcium and lead, fluoride for calcium, magnesium and lead, ferrocyanide for zinc and copper and 8-hydroxyquinoline for many heavy metals.

2. **Masking by complex formation**: Masking agents must produce more stable complexes with the interfering metal ions under analysis.

Demasking: It is a process in which the masked substance regains its ability to enter into a particular reaction. This enables us to determine a series of metal ions in one solution containing many cations. Examples of using masking and demasking reagents in complexometry are the assay of a mixture of three metals-copper, cadmium and calcium. Following method of analysis is utilized:

1. Direct titration of the mixture with EDTA gives the sum of the three methods.

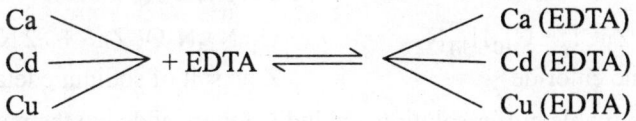

2. Copper and cadmium may be masked with the addition of cyanide to the solution leaving only the calcium ion.

3. When formaldehyde or chloral hydrate is added to the cyanide containing mixture only cadmium is demasked and the EDTA titrates the sum of calcium and cadmium. In this manner the concentration of all three ions are determined by three individual titrations.

Step (1): All the three metals are titrated.
Step (2): Only the Ca^{2+} metal is titrated.

$$Cu + cyanide\ ion \longrightarrow Cu\text{-cyanide complex}$$

$$Cd + cyanide\ ion \longrightarrow Cd\text{-cyanide complex}$$

$$Ca + cyanide\ ion \longrightarrow No\ reaction$$

$$Ca + (EDTA) \longrightarrow Ca\ (EDTA)$$

Step (3): The Cd and Cu metals are titrated

$$Cu\text{-cyanide complex} \longrightarrow No\ reaction$$
$$+ CH_2O \text{ (Formic acid)}$$

$$Cd\text{-cyanide complex} \longrightarrow Cd + CH_2CN$$

$$+ CH_2O \text{ (Formic acid)}$$
$$\text{(Masking agent)}$$

Preparation and standardization of 0.05 m disodium edetate solution: It is based on titration of the prepared disodium edetate solution with a standard zinc chloride solution prepared from a known weight of granulated zinc.

$$\underset{\text{Zinc}}{Zn} + 2\,HCl \longrightarrow \underset{\text{Zinc chloride}}{ZnCl_2} + H_2$$

$$\underset{\text{Zinc chloride}}{ZnCl_2 + C_{10}H_{14}N_2} \longrightarrow \underset{\text{Zinc salt of sodium edetate}}{C_{10}N_{14}N_2O_8\,Zn} + 2\,NaCl$$

A suitable buffer solution and indicator are added to the metal ion solution and the solution titrated with standard disodium edetate until the indicator just changes color. A blank titration may by performed by omitting the sample.

Preparation: Dissolve disodium edetate (18.61 g) in sufficient amount of water to produce 1000 ml. Mordant black 11 mixture is used as an indicator in ammonia buffer.

Procedure: Dissolve granulated zinc (0.8 g) in dilute hydrochloric acid (12 ml) and bromine water (0.1 ml) by gentle warming. Boil to remove excess of bromine, cool and add neutralize with 2M sodium hydroxide solutions. Dilute the solution with water (150 ml) and add sufficient buffer (pH 10.0) to dissolve edetate solution until the solution turns green.

Factor: Each ml of 0.05 M disodium edentate is equivalent to 0.000654 g of zinc.

(A) Determination of Magnesium (Mg) By Titration With EDTA

Many metal ions react with electron pair donors to form coordination compounds or complex ions. The formation of a particular class of coordination compounds, called chelates, are especially well suited for quantitative methods. A chelate is formed when a metal ion coordinates with two (or more) donor groups of a single ligand. Tertiary amine compounds, such as ethylenediamine tetraacetic acid (EDTA), are widely used for the formation of chelates.

Complexometric titrations with EDTA have been reported for the analysis of nearly all metal ions. Because EDTA has four acidic protons, the formation of metal-ion/EDTA complexes is dependent upon the pH. For the titration of Mg^{2+}, one must buffer the solution to a pH of 10 so that complex formation will be quantitative. The reaction of Mg^{2+} with EDTA may be expressed as:

$$Mg^{2+} + H_2Y_2^- = MgY^{2-} + 2H^+$$

The end point of the titration is determined by the addition of Eriochrome black T, which forms a colored chelate with Mg^{2+} and undergoes a color change when the Mg^{2+} is released to form a chelate with EDTA. While it is possible to achieve relatively good results by titration with EDTA prepared directly from the solid, better results should be obtained when the EDTA is standardized against a solution containing a known amount of metal ion.

Reagents Used

1. EDTA: 1000 ml has been prepared by dissolving 70.0 g of NH_4Cl in 325 ml of deionized water, adding 568 ml of conc. ammonia and diluting to 1000 ml

2. Eriochrome Black T

3. 6 M HCl

4. 1 M NH_4OH

5. Standard Zn solution

Accurately weighed (1.3g) of pure zinc has been dissolved in a small volume (15 ml) of 6M HCl. The dissolve zinc was quantitatively transferred to a volumetric flask and diluted to the mark. This 0.01 M solution serves to standardize the EDTA solution.

Procedure: Dilute the unknown sample to 100 ml exactly and mix thoroughly. Transfer exactly 10 ml of the unknown solution into 3 or 4 conical flasks. Add 15 ml of pH 10 buffer in the hood and 20 or 25 ml of distilled, deionized water to each flask. Add few crystals of Eriochrome black T indicator to produce a light, wine-red color. Titrate each solution with the standardized EDTA solution to a clear blue color.

(B) Determination of Calcium by Titration With a Chelating Ligand EDTA

Ethylene diamine tetra acetic acid (EDTA) contains six sites that can be protonated. Since EDTA itself is quite insoluble in water, the disodium salt is normally used to make EDTA solutions. To form the strongest complexes, EDTA solutions are usually buffered in a region that ensures that protonation reactions do not compete with the complexation reaction. The important species in solution are generally H_2Y^{2-} and HY^{3-}.

$$Ca^{2+} + HY^{2-} = CaY^{2-} + H^+$$

Since EDTA forms very strong complexes with most metal ions with a charge greater than +2, procedures designed to "mask" or complex impurity ions are often used. In this experiment, however, relatively pure calcium carbonate is used, so that masking reagents are not needed. The overall procedure to be used involves the standardization of an EDTA solution by titration with a known amount of calcium followed by using the calibrated solution to determine an unknown amount of calcium.

Procedure

A. Preparation of Primary Standard Calcium Solution

1. The primary standard calcium carbonate should be dried at 150°C for at least 1 hour.
2. Prepare a calcium standard solution by accurately weighing 0.35 - 0.4 g of standard calcium carbonate and quantitatively transferring the solid to a 250 ml beaker.
3. Place the beaker in the hood and add 6M HCl drop wise until the sample completely dissolves. Make the volume up to about 50 ml with distilled water.
4. Gently boil the solution for a few minutes to expel excess CO_2 being careful not to lose any of the solution.
5. Allow the solution to cool and add two drops of methyl red indicator.
6. Add drops of 6 M NaOH until the methyl red indicator turns yellow (the yellow may be difficult to see but there is no trace of red). Any flocculent precipitate that forms may indicate that too much NaOH has been added. Add a drop or two of HCl to dissolve the precipitate.
7. Carefully rinse the beaker with distilled water into a 100 ml volumetric flask to quantitatively transfer all of the calcium solution. Dilute to the mark in the volumetric flask. Mix the solution carefully before continuing.

B. Unknown Calcium Samples (Treat in the Same Manner as the CaCO₃ Standard)

1. Use the unknown calcium samples from the previous week's experiment and dry in a weighing bottle in the oven at 150°C for at least 30 minutes.
2. Be sure to record the unknown number in your laboratory notebook and the laboratory sample log book.
3. Remove the unknown from the oven and allow it to cool before weighing.
4. Estimate the number of grams of unknown required to use about 35 ml of your standardized EDTA solution.
5. Place the flask in the hood and add 6M HCl drop wise until the sample dissolves. Some samples may have a trace of very fine insoluble silica (sand) that appears transparent upon close observation. Make the volume up to about 50 ml with distilled water.
6. Gently boil the solution for a few minutes to expel excess CO_2 being careful not to lose any of the solution.
7. Allow the solution to cool and add two drops of methyl red indicator.
8. Add drops of 6 M NaOH until the methyl red indicator turns yellow.
9. Any flocculent precipitate that forms may indicate that too much NaOH has been added. Add a drop or two of HCl to dissolve the precipitate.
10. Carefully rinse the beaker with distilled water into a 100 ml volumetric flask to quantitatively transfer all of the calcium solution. Dilute to the mark in the volumetric flask. Mix the solution carefully before continuing.
11. Pipette a 10 ml aliquot of the calcium unknown into a 250 ml Erlenmeyer flask and add 15 ml of the ammonium hydroxide-ammonium chloride (NH_4OH-NH_4Cl) buffer.
12. Add 10 drops of calmagite indicator.
13. Add enough distilled water to have a total volume of 75-100 ml in the Erlenmeyer flask.

14. Titrate from the initial wine red color to an end point of sky blue.
15. Titrations should take between 30 and 40 ml of EDTA titrant to minimize the burette volume error.
16. Obtain at least three good reproducible titrations. The results should agree to within ±1%. Calculate the amount of calcium in the unknown at this point.

C. Determination of Total Hardness of Water by Complexometry

EDTA is used as a complexing reagent and it forms soluble complexes with metal ions like calcium and magnesium. End point in this titration is detected by color change of the indicator Eriochrome black T. The stability of the complex and color change of the indicator depends upon the pH of the titrating medium. Hence the solution to be titrated must be well buffered by ammonium hydroxide-ammonium chloride (NH_4OH-NH_4Cl) buffer solution of pH- 10. at the end point, the concentration of metal ion decreases abruptly. A metal ion indicator forms a complex with metal ion.

$$M^{2+} + HIn^{2-} \longrightarrow MIn^- + H^+$$

Where HIn^{2-} shows indicator form at a particular pH.

However, metal ion indicator complexes are usually less stable than the metal-EDTA complexes. The indicator releases the metal ions at the end point and this shows a color change. In this titration, in the presence of metal ions, Eriochrome black T forma a wine red complex. At the end point, when the metal ions are completely complexed with EDTA, the color changes to blue (of the free indicator)

$$\underset{\text{Winered}}{MIn^-} + H_2Y^{2-} \longrightarrow MY^{2-} + \underset{\text{Colorless blue}}{HIn^{2-} + H^+}$$

The Ca-Mg-EDTA complexes are stable at pH 8–10, the pH of the solution during the titrations must be maintained at 10 (by NH_4OH-NH_4Cl buffer). Hence Ca^{2+} ions do not form a sufficiently stable complex with Eriochrome black-T, Mg-EDTA complex is added to the titration flask; if the sample either does not contain sufficient Mg^{2+} ions (or does not contain all) to produce a sharp color change at the end point. Chemical reactions may be shown as:

$$Ca^{2+} + H_2Y^{2-} \longrightarrow CaY^{2-} + 2H^+$$

$$Ca^{2+} + H_2Y^{2-} \longrightarrow MgY^{2-} + 2H^+$$

$$Mg^{2+} + HIn^{2-} \longrightarrow MgIn^- + H^+$$

$$MIn^- + H_2Y^{2-} \longrightarrow MY^{2-} + HIn^{2-} + H^+$$

Wine red   Colorless   blue   at the end point

From the above reactions, it is clear that one mole of the disodium salt of EDTA reacts with one mole of Ca^{2+} / Mg^{2+} ions. Therefore, the molarities are related as:

$$M_1V_1 / M_2V_2 = 1/1 \text{ or } M_1 V_1 = M_2 V_2$$

Where M_1 / M_2 = Molarities of EDTA salt and metal-ions solution respectively and

V_1, V_2 = Their volumes, respectively.

Procedure: Rinse and fill the burette with the 0.01M EDTA solution. Pipette out 60 ml of the water sample into a 250 ml conical flask, add 2 ml of the buffer solution.0.5 ml of Mg-EDTA complex solution (mandatory) and five drops of the indicator. The color of the titration mixture at this stage must be wine red. Titrate with 0.01M EDTA from the burette with constant swirling. The solution should be stirred thoroughly and the EDTA solution added slowly drop wise near the end point. The color changes from wine red thoroughly purple to a clear blue at the end point.

Calculations

Let W be the weight of EDTA dissolved in 250 cm^3.

Therefore, the molarity of EDTA solution = 4W/372.3 = ... mol/dm^3

Volume of EDTA used= V_1 ml and volume of water sample = 60 ml

Molarity of Ca^{2+}/Mg^{2+} in water sample = M_2

$M_2 = M_1V_1/V_2$ mol/dm^3

Total hardness of the sample in mg of $CaCO_3/dm^3$ of water = $M_2 \times 100 \times 1000$. (Molar mass of $CaCO_3$ = 100)

D. Determination of Bismuth by Direct EDTA Titration

Procedure: Accurately weigh about 5 g of bismuth subnitrate $Bi(NO_3)_3.5H_2O$ or bismuth carbonate $(BiO)_2 CO_3.\frac{1}{2}H_2O$, first add a little HNO_3 and then deionized water, shake to dissolve and make up with the water up to 1000 ml. This is about 0.01 M bismuth solution. Pipette out 25 ml of the Bi^{3+} ion solution into a 500 ml conical flask and dilute to 150 ml of water. If necessary, adjust the pH to about 1 by the careful addition of dilute aqueous ammonia solution or of dilute HNO_3 and take the help of pH meter. Add 5 drops of xylenol orange indicator. Titrate with 0.01 M EDTA solution until the intense red color of the indicator starts diluting. When this condition is reached titrate drop wise, swirl the mixture, wait and proceed until the indicator changes to yellow (end point). Repeat the titration at least three times more to fix the titre valve.

1 mole of EDTA = 1 mole Bi^{3+} ion

6.8 Applications of Complexometric Titrations

A number of pharmaceutical substances can be assayed by official methods employed sodium edetate titration.

1. Assay of Calcium Carbonate (CaCO₃)

I.P.Limit: Calcium carbonate contains not less than 98% and not more than the equivalent of 100.5% of $CaCO_3$ calculated with reference to the dried substances.

Theory: Calcium carbonate forms complex with 0.05 M sodium edetate. Calcon mixture is added as an indicator. It is pink in color in the presence of calcium salt (calcium-indicator complex) but blue in color in the absence of calcium carbonate, hence, at the end point blue color is obtained. Indicator is added towards the end of the titration. Sodium hydroxide is added to maintain the alkaline pH.

Procedure: Weigh accurately calcium carbonate (0.1 g) and dissolve in dilute hydrochloric acid (3 ml) in water (10 ml). Boil for 10 minutes, cool, dilute to 50 ml with water. Titrate with 0.05 M disodium edetate, then add sodium hydroxide (8 ml) and calcon mixture (0.1 g) and continue the titration until the color of the solution changes from pink to full blue color.

Factor: Each ml of 0.05 M disodium edetate is equivalent to 0.0050048 g of $CaCO_3$

2. Assay of Magnesium Sulphate (MgSO₄)

I.P.Limit: Magnesium sulphate contains not less than 99% and not more than the equivalent of 100% of $MgSO_4$, calculated with reference to the ignited substances.

Theory: Magnesium sulphate forms complex with 0.05 M sodium edetate. Mordant black II mixture is added as an indicator. It is pink in color in the presence of magnesium salt (magnesium-indicator complex) but blue in color in the absence of magnesium sulphate, hence, at the end point blue color is obtained. Indicator is added towards the end of the titration.

Procedure: Weigh accurately magnesium sulphate (0.3 g) and dilute to 50 ml of water. Add strong ammonia-ammonium chloride solution (10 ml) and titrate with 0.05 M disodium edetate using mordant black II (0.1 g) as an indicator and continue the titration until the color of the solution changes from pink to blue.

Factor: Each ml of 0.05 M disodium edetate is equivalent to 0.00602 g of $MgSO_4$.

EXERCISES

1. What are complexometric titrations? Discuss in detail the principal involved.

2. Describe types of EDTA complexometric titration.

3. Write a note on masking and demasking agents. What are its advantages?

4. What is the difference between complexometry and volumetric analysis?

5. Explain the preparation and standardization of 0.05 M disodium edetate.

6. Write a note on complexometric titration curve.

7. Give the theory involved in complexometric titration.

8. Mention some indicators used in complexometric titrations.

9. Discuss the effect of pH on assays in complexometric titrations.

10. Write a note on theory involved in complexometric titrations.

11. Give the determination of total hardness of water by complexometry

12. Explain the determination of calcium by titrating agent like EDTA.

13. Write a note on complexometric titration with EDTA.

14. Give the determination of magnesium by complexometry.

15. Describe the assay procedure of ;
    (i) Calcium carbonate
    (ii) Magnesium sulphate
    (iii) Calcium gluconate
    (iv) Bismuth carbonate
    (v) Bismuth sub nitrate.

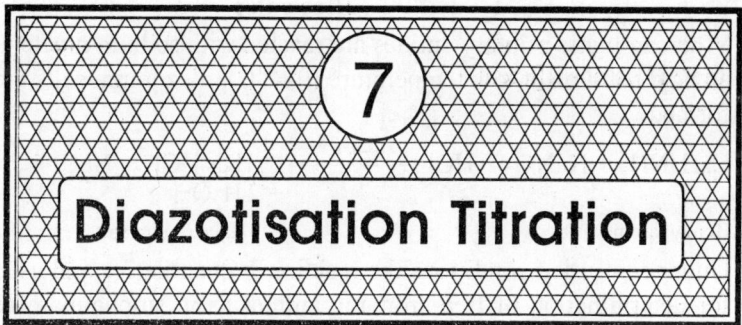

Diazotisation Titration

Diazotisation is a reaction that converts an $-NH_2$ group connected to a phenyl ring to a diazonium salt ($Ar-N_2^+X^-$). The nitrous acid provides NO^+ which replaces a hydrogen on the $-NH_3^+$ group to produce $-NH_2NO^+$ and water; a second water is eliminated to produce the $-N_2^+$ group.

In diazotisation titrations or sodium nitrite titrations, the substance containing primary aromatic amino group is converted into the respective diazonium salt by treating with sodium nitrite at low temperature in the presence of hydrochloric acid. In general, aromatic primary amino moiety ($Ar-NH_2$), as present in sulpha drugs and other pharmaceutical preparations, e.g., sodium and calcium aminosalicylate, isocarboxazid, primaquine phosphate and dapsone, react with sodium nitrite in an acidic medium to yield the diazonium salts as expressed below;

$$ArNH_2 + NaNO_2 + HCl \xrightarrow{0-4°C} ArN_2^+Cl^- + NaCl + 2H_2O$$

Amine   sodium nitrite   Diazonium salt

At the end point, a drop of nitrous acid (formed from sodium nitrite ($NaNO_2$) in acid medium) reacts with starch iodide paper and gives blue color due to liberation of iodine.

$$2HI + 2HNO_2 \longrightarrow I_2 + 2NO\uparrow + 2H_2O$$

Nitrous acid

$$I_2 \xrightarrow{\text{Starch}} \text{Blue color}$$

When aromatic primary amines are reacted with sodium nitrite in an acid solution at low temperature ($0-4^\circ C$), diazonium salts are formed.

$$C_6H_5NH_2 + NaNO_2 + HCl \xrightarrow{0-4^\circ C} C_6H_5N_2^+Cl^- + NaCl + 2H_2O$$

Benzyl amine   Diazonium salt

Under controlled conditions the reaction is quantitative and used for determination of free aromatic amines as in sulphanilamide and other sulpha drugs. The presence of a small excess of nitrous acid indicates the end point which is detected using starch–iodide paper as an external indicator.

$$KI + HCl \longrightarrow HI + KCl$$

$$2HI + 2HNO_2 \longrightarrow I_2 + 2NO + 2H_2O$$

The liberated iodine reacts with starch to form a blue color complex. The end point may also be detected electrometrically.

7.1 Conditions Iinvolved in Diazotisation of Different Amines

Depending upon the properties of the analysed amines the condition of diazotisation titration may vary although the procedure remains the same. The most important conditions are:

(1) Rate of titration: Different amino compounds react with nitrous acid at different rates when titration is conducted. Therefore sodium nitrite added needs time to change into nitrous acid and enter into the reaction with amine without accumulating in solution under test. Amines are classified as rapidly or slowly diazotisable depending upon the rate of conversion into diazo compounds.

- Rapidly diazotisable amino compounds include compound sulpha group, nitro group or carbonyl group containing aromatic compounds besides the amino group, e.g., isomeric nitro aniline, sulphanilic acid and anthralinic acid.
- Slowly diazotisable amino compounds are those which do not contain any substituent group other than amino group or along with amino they may contain $-CH_3$ or $-OH$ group, e.g., isomeric amino phenol, aniline and toluidine.

The rate of diazotisation can be increased by adding KBr to solution under test containing amine and inorganic acid. In case of slowly diazotisable amino compounds for detecting the end point sufficient time about 5-10 minutes should be given to solution under test so that the last portion of nitrite could fully react with amine. If the test for end point determination is made immediately after titration, the nitrous acid that has not get enabled into reactions with amine will be taken for excess acid indicating that the end point has reached. By efficient stirring and slow addition of sodium nitrite ($NaNO_2$) solution, a large excess of sodium nitrite ($NaNO_2$) is not allowed to build up. It is also suggested that burette tip is placed below the surface of heating nitrous acid.

(2) Effect of Temperature: Diazo compounds are unstable and readily decomposed at higher temperature. This can lead to side reactions and give wrong results. To eliminate this, titrations are carried out at low temperature. The optimum temperature of most amines is $15-20\,^{\circ}C$ where they are relatively stable diazo compounds. Amines that form unstable diazo compounds are titrated at temperature of $0-4\,^{\circ}C$.

7.2 End Point Determination

The end point determination in diazotisation titration is done by two important methods, viz;

1. Visual end point determination method.
2. Electrometric end point determination method.

1. Visual end point determination method: When aromatic primary amines are reacted with sodium nitrite in acid solution at low temperature ($0-4^{\circ}C$), diazonium salts are formed.

$$C_6H_5NH_2 + NaNO_2 + HCl \xrightarrow{\;0-4^{\circ}C\;} C_6H_5N_2^+Cl^- + NaCl + 2H_2O$$

Benzylamine   Sodium nitrite

Diazonium salt

Under controlled conditions the reaction is quantitative and used for determination of free aromatic amines as in sulphanilamide and other sulpha drugs. Observation of the end point depends upon the detection of small amount of nitrous acid which is present in the solution as excess. This can be demonstrated visually using **starch iodide paper or paste** as external indicator.

$$2\,HI + 2\,HNO_2 \longrightarrow I_2 + 2\,NO + 2\,H_2O$$

$$I_2 \xrightarrow{\text{Starch}} \text{Blue color}$$

Method: Weigh accurately about 1.25 g of sample, dissolve in glacial acetic acid (50 ml) and warm gently, if necessary. Add cold water (175 ml) and cool below 10°C, add hydrochloric acid (10 ml) and slowly titrate with 0.1 M $NaNO_2$ solution at a temperature below 10°C until a drop of the solution immediately gives a blue color when drawn quickly by means of a fine rod across the surface of a starch iodide paper.

The titration is complete when the end point is reproducible after the titrated solution has been allowed to stand for 6 minutes.

2. Electrometric end point determination method: End point may be detected electrometrically using a pair of bright platinum electrode immersed in the titration liquid. Electrode polarization occurs when a small voltage of 30-50 mV is applied across the electrodes and no current flows through the sensitive galvanometer included in the circuit, during the course of titration. Liberation of excess of nitrous acid at the point depolarizes the electrodes, current flows in the galvanometer and the permanent deflection of galvanometer needle is observed. This is known as **dead-stop end point.** In such method the electrode used must be cleaned otherwise the end point is sluggish.

Cleaning of electrode can be accomplished by immersing the electrode in boiling nitric acid containing a little ferric chloride for about 30 seconds and then washing with water. A blank determination is necessary; the difference between the two titrations represents the volume of sodium nitrite solution equivalent to the aromatic amine.

Method: Weigh accurately about 0.5 g of sample, dissolve in glacial acetic acid (10 ml) and warm gently, if necessary. Add cold water (75 ml) and cool below 10°C, add hydrochloric acid (10 ml). Insert a pair of bright platinum electrode into the solution, connected through a sensitive galvanometer and a suitable potentiometer to a 2V battery in such a way so as to produce a potential drop of between 30–50 mV across the electrodes. Titrate slowly with 0.1 M $NaNO_2$ solution with continuous stirring until a permanent deflection of galvanometer needle is observed at the end point.

7.3 Applications of Diazotisation Titrations

A number of pharmaceutical substances can be assayed by official methods employed sodium nitrite titration. Important applications of sodium nitrite titrations includes the analysis of following compounds:

1. Sulphadiazine
2. Sulphanilamide
3. Dapsone
4. Sodium aminosalicylate
5. Benzocaine
6. Procaine HCl
7. Calcium aminosalicylate
8. Sulphacetamide tablets
9. Sulphacetamide eye ointment
10. Succinyl sulphathiazole, and
11. Isocarboxazid

7.4 Assays in Diazotisation Titrations

A few typical examples are described below to get an in-depth knowledge about sodium nitrite titrations.

1. Assay of Sodium Aminosalicylate

Theory: Nitrous acid is formed from sodium nitrite in acidic medium which diazotizes sulphanilamide to form the diazonium salt. At the end point, a slight excess of nitrous acid reacts with starch iodide paper to give the blue color. Treatment of sodium aminosalicylate ($C_7H_6NNaO_3$) with sodium nitrite forms a diazonium salt.

Reaction involved

$$NaNO_2 + HCl \longrightarrow HNO_2 + NaCl$$

Sodium nitrite — Nitrous acid

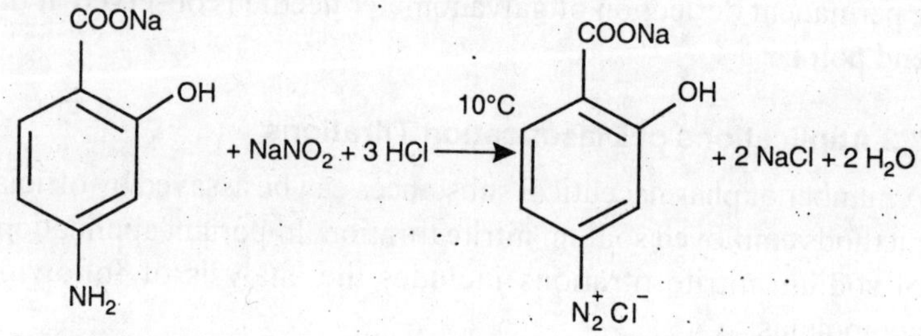

Sodium aminosalicylate — Diazonium salt of sodium aminosalicylate

Fig. 7.1: Formation of sodium aminosalicylate diazonium salt.

Procedure: Weigh accurately about 0.25 g of sample and dissolve in glacial acetic acid (50 ml), warm gently, if necessary. Add cold water (175 ml) and cool below 10°C, add hydrochloric acid (10 ml) and slowly titrate with 0.1 M sodium nitrite at a temperature below 10°C until a drop of the solution immediately gives a blue color when drawn quickly by means of a fine rod across the surface of a starch iodide paper.

The titration is complete when the end point is reproducible after the titrated solution has been allowed to stand for 6 minutes. The end point may also be determined by electrometric method.

Factor: 1 ml 0.1 M $NaNO_2$ = 0.01752 g of C_7H_6

2. Assay of Dapsone [Electrometrically]

Preparation of 0.1 M $NaNO_2$: Weigh accurately 7.5 g of sodium nitrite and add sufficient distilled water to produce 1 litre in a 1000 ml volumetric flask.

Standardization of 0.1 M $NaNO_2$ with $KMnO_4$: Take 25 ml of potassium permanganate ($KMnO_4$) in a 100 ml conical flask; add 30 ml of water and 4.5 ml of concentrated H_2SO_4. Shake and heat the solution to maintain the temperature between 40-60°C and slowly titrate the solution with 0.1 M $NaNO_2$ solution with continuous stirring until a violet color is observed at the end point.

Factor: 1 ml 0.1 M KMnO$_4$ ≡ 0.034 g of NaNO$_3$.

Reaction involved

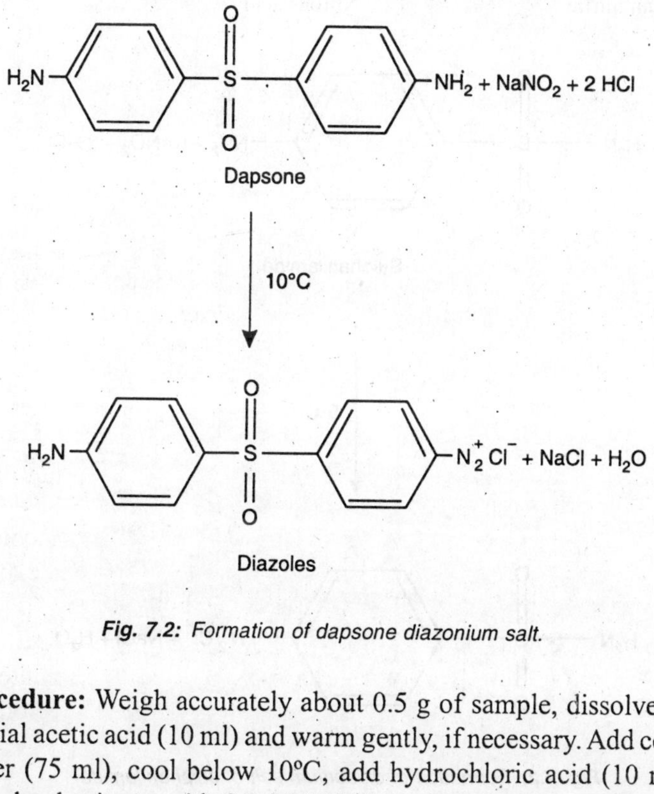

Dapsone

10°C

Diazoles

Fig. 7.2: *Formation of dapsone diazonium salt.*

Procedure: Weigh accurately about 0.5 g of sample, dissolve in glacial acetic acid (10 ml) and warm gently, if necessary. Add cold water (75 ml), cool below 10°C, add hydrochloric acid (10 ml) and slowly titrate with 0.1 M NaNO$_2$ solution with continuous stirring until a permanent deflection of galvanometer needle is observed at the end point.

Factor: 1 ml 0.1 M NaNO$_2$ ≡ 0.01242 g of C$_{12}$H$_{12}$N$_2$O$_2$S.

3. Assay of Sulphanilamide

Theory: Nitrous acid is formed from sodium nitrite in acidic medium which diazotizes sulphanilamide to form the diazonium salt. At the end point, a slight excess of nitrous acid reacts with starch iodide paper to give the blue color.

Reaction involved

$$NaNO_2 \;+\; HCl \;\longrightarrow\; HNO_2 \;+\; NaCl$$

Sodium nitrite   Nitrous acid

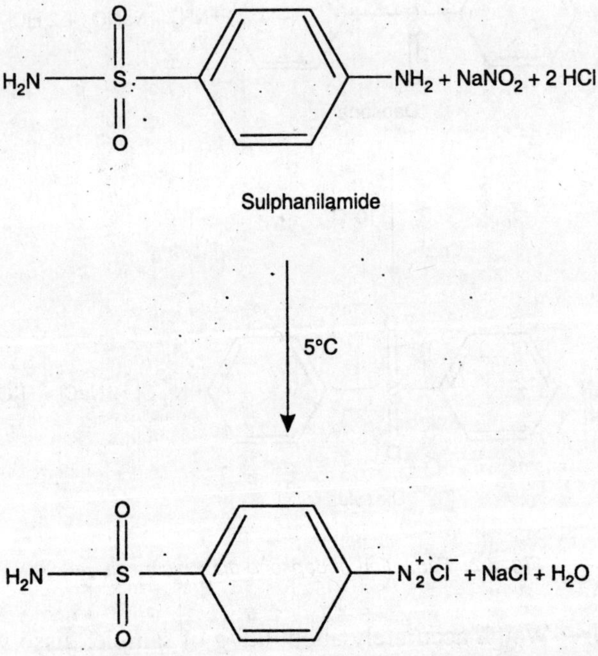

Fig. 7.2: Formation of diazonium salt of sulphanilamide

Procedure: Weigh accurately about 1 g of sulphanilamide and dissolve in hydrochloric acid (40 ml) and water (100 ml). The solutions is cooled to about 5 °C and slowly titrate with 0.1 M sodium nitrite until a drop of the solution immediately gives a blue color when drawn quickly by means of a fine rod across the surface of a starch iodide paper. The titration is complete when the end point is reproducible after the titrated solution has been allowed to stand for 1 minute.

Factor: 1 ml 0.1 M $NaNO_2$ = 0.01722 g of sulphanilamide.

EXERCISES

1. What are sodium nitrite titrations? Discuss in detail the principal involved.
2. What are the differences between diazotisation titrations and complexometric titrations?
3. Discuss the preparation and standardization of 0.1N sodium nitrite.
4. Give the theory involved in sodium nitrite titration.
5. Mention some indicators used in sodium nitrite titrations.
6. Write a note on end point determination in diazotisation titration
7. Describe conditions involved in diazotisation of different amines.
8. Give the assay procedure of
   - (i) Sulphanilamide
   - (ii) Dapsone
   - (iii) Sodium aminosalicylate

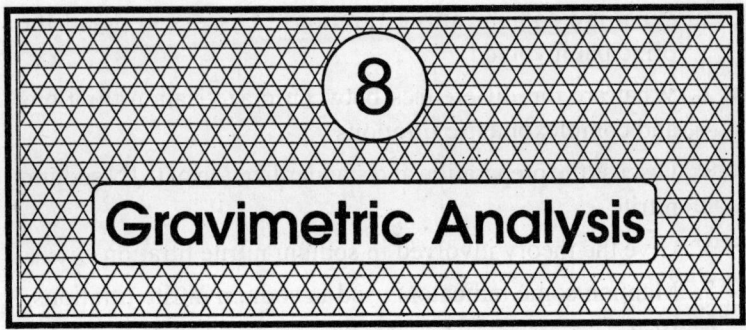

8
Gravimetric Analysis

Precipitation is a process of producing a separable solid phase within a liquid medium. In analytical chemistry, precipitation is widely used to effect the separation of a solid phase in an aqueous solution. For example, the addition of silver nitrate to an aqueous solution of sodium chloride results in the formation of insoluble silver chloride. Quite often, one of the components in the solution is thus completely separated in a relatively pure form. It can then be isolated from the solution phase by filtration or centrifugation, and determined by weighing. This procedure is known as *gravimetric analysis*.

Precipitation may also be used merely to effect partial or complete separation of a substance for purposes other than that of gravimetric analysis. Such purposes might involve either the isolation of a relatively pure substance or the removal of undesirable components of the solution.

A component can be separated from a solution by determining from the solubility product constant. It is obtained by determining the quantity of the dissolved substance present in a known amount of a saturated solution. This value is known as the *solubility*. The solubility can be drastically altered by adding to the solution any of the ions that make up the precipitate, for example, by adding varying quantities of either silver nitrate or sodium chloride to a saturated solution of silver chloride. Although solubility can be altered over a wide range, the solubility product itself remains practically constant over this same range.

Various techniques may be employed in order to reduce contamination by foreign ions. Precipitation from dilute solution is often effective. Heating the reaction mixture speeds recrystallization processes by which incorporated foreign ions may be returned to the solution phase. Precipitation from homogeneous solution results in the slow formation of large crystals of small surface area and, hence, lessens co-precipitation. If all these methods fail to reduce adequately the quantity of foreign ions incorporated in the solid phase, the precipitate is dissolved and reprecipitated by the previous procedure.

8.1 Definitions and Classification

Gravimetric titration or analysis means "quantitative analysis by weighing". It involves the separation of the constituents to be estimated in the form of an insoluble precipitate. Gravimetric analysis is a modification of precipitation reaction in which the insoluble precipitate formed is washed to free it from all impurities, dried and weighed either as such or ignited to leave a residue of some other compound which is then weighed. Now from its weight and known composition, the amount of the constituent in the given sample is calculated, e.g., determination of chlorine content in a sample of NaCl.

The various forms of gravimetric analysis are:

1. Electrogravimetry involves electrolysis and the material deposited on one of the electrodes is weighed.

2. Thermogravimetry (TG) records the change in weight as a function of temperature.

3. Differential Thermal Analysis (DTA) records the difference in temperature between a test substance and an inert reference material.

4. Differential Scanning Colorimetry (DSC) records the energy needed to establish a zero temperature difference between a test substance and a reference material.

In the determination of silver nitrate ($AgNO_3$) sample suppose silver ion (Ag) is the constituent to be determined. Therefore, it is separated from other components of sample in a form of insoluble complex or precipitate by adding suitable precipitating agent (precipitant) shown as;

$$AgNO_3 \quad + \quad KCNS \quad \longrightarrow \quad AgCNS\downarrow \quad + \quad KNO_3$$

Silver	Potassium	Silver	Potassium
nitrate	thiocyanate	thiocyanate	nitrate
(analyte)	(precipitant)	(precipitate)	

Now AgCNS precipitate is washed, dried and weighed and the determination are involving weight by subtraction method as:
  (i) Weight of sample taken for analysis = x.
 (ii) Weight of the pure precipitate containing the constituent of the sample to be determined = y.
(iii) Weight of constituent = Weight of sample taken-Weight of precipitate.

$$(z) = x - y$$

Chlorine content may be determined by various methods on the basis of this reaction. For example, the precipitated silver chloride (AgCl) can be filtered off, washed thoroughly, carefully dried and accurately weighed. From the weight of silver chloride (AgCl) precipitate and its formula, it is easy to calculate the chlorine content. Thus, in the analysis of 0.0536 g of sodium chloride (NaCl) the precipitate weighed 0.1290 g, since one gram-molecule (i.e., 143.3 g) silver chloride (AgCl) contains one gram atom (i.e., 34.45 g) chloride ion (Cl), we can write:

143.3 g AgCl contains 35.45 g of Cl

$$x \text{ g AgCl contains } \frac{35.45}{143.3} \text{ g of Cl}$$

Therefore, 0.1290 g AgCl contains $\dfrac{35.45}{143.3} \times 0.1290$ g of Cl = 0.03192 g Cl.

Since all the chlorine is originally present in the weighed samples of common salt (NaCl), the percentage chlorine content of the latter is easily found,

$$0.0536 \text{ g NaCl contains } 0.03192 \text{ g of Cl}$$
$$100 \text{ g AgCl contains } y \text{ g of Cl}$$

$$y = \frac{0.03192}{0.0536} \times 100 = 59.6\%$$

8.2 Solubility Product

The process of gravimetric precipitation titration is completely based on the concepts of solubility product. Let us consider a dissociation of slightly soluble salt AB.

In solution it will exist in equilibrium with its dissociation ions as in

$$AB \rightleftharpoons A^+ + B^-$$

Applying law of mass action.

$$K = \frac{\left[A^+\right]\left[B^-\right]}{AB}$$

The concentration of the AB in the solution remains constant in the presence of undissolved AB, i.e.

$$K_{Sp} = \frac{\left[A^+\right]\left[B^-\right]}{AB} \quad \text{or} \quad K_{Sp} \equiv [A^+] + [B^-]$$

Where K_{Sp} is constant at constant temperature and is called solubility product of salt [AB], and is defined as the maximum product of the concentration of its constituent ions in its solution.

$[A^+]$ and $[B^-]$ = Ionic concentration in saturated solution.

If the ionic product or concentration is greater (>) than $K_{Sp} \rightarrow$ precipitation will occur.

If the ionic product or concentration is lesser (<) than $K_{Sp} \rightarrow$ precipitation do not occur.

If the ionic product or concentration is equal (=) to $K_{Sp} \rightarrow$ solution remains saturated.

Therefore, lesser the solubility product, easier will be the precipitation.

Based on solubility product of excess of Ag^+ ions are added to the saturated solutions of silver chloride (AgCl) in water, the ionic product of $[Ag^+][Cl^-]$ is exceeded and consequently some silver chloride (AgCl) will be precipitated.

Table 8.1: *Comparison between volumetric and gravimetric analysis*

Volumetric analysis	Gravimetric analysis
Quantitative analysis by measuring volume of solutions of the interacting substances.	Quantitative analysis by measuring the weight of constituent to be determined
Rapid and less time consuming	Slower process and time consuming
Possibility of errors are large, hence less accurate	Precipitates are cheered from all impurities hence maximizing the possibility of errors are less and high level of accuracy is determined
Calibration of apparatus required for determination of % purity	An absolute method involves direct measurement without any form calibrations.
Involve relatively small samples.	Involve relatively large samples.

8.3 Steps of Gravimetric Analysis

1. **Sampling**: An ideal sample would be identical in all its properties with the bulk of the material from which it is taken. Cost of test, value of product, end use of products, accuracy of test method and nature of materials used are considered in this step.

2. **Dissolution of the sample**: To dissolve the sample analyte, take a clean beaker and transfer the weighed sample completely to the beaker. Add sufficient water or acid or alkali to the sample to get a clear solution. If the heating is necessary for dissolution, then heat the solution on a water bath with asbestos gauze to form the clear solution.

3. **Precipitation**: For the ideal precipitant, it should react with analyte to form the precipitate which can be easily filtered; washed free of contaminating impurities, low solubility, stable and should have constant known composition after drying.

4. **Testing the completeness of precipitation reaction:** To achieve the complete precipitation, the precipitating agent is added in slight excess. In the procedure, during the formation of precipitate, it is allowed to settle down and then few-drops of precipitating agent are added slowly through a rod to the upper supernatant liquid. If precipitation occurs at this stage, the precipitation is not complete, and more reagents should be added to the solution. But if no precipitation occurs at the stage, precipitation is complete and there is no need of adding more precipitating reagent. It is always advisable to check the completeness of precipitation before the digestion and filtration.

5. **Digestion:** Digestion is generally carried out at higher temperature to speed up the process but in some cases it is done at room temperature. It improves the purity and rate of filtration of precipitate. The surface adsorption is also minimized.

6. **Filtration:** In this operation, precipitate is separated from mother liquor. Various types of filter media's are used for this purpose.

7. **Washing of precipitate:** After filtering the precipitate, the impurities on the surface of precipitate can be removed by washing of the precipitate. Ideal washing solution should have no solvent action on the precipitate but should dissolve foreign matter easily. Many precipitates are not washed with water, but with washing solution.

8. **Drying and ignition of precipitate:** The main objective of drying is to convert the precipitate into weighed form having constant composition. It is heated to remove water and to remove the adsorbed electrolyte from washing solution. Drying or ignition process will depend on nature of precipitates and the filtering media used for the purpose. Drying is the term used when temperature is below 250°C and ignition above 250°C and below 1200°C. Ignition is done by heating with appropriate burner or crucible can be placed in electrically heated muffle furnace.

9. **Weighing and calculations:** The residue after drying is cooled to room temperature in a desicator and then weighed accurately on the analytical balance to find out the weighed form.

The calculations are generally made in terms of percentage

$$\% A = \frac{gA}{g\,(\text{Sample})} \times 100$$

$g\,A$ = grams of analyte

g sample = grams of sample taken for the analysis.

By knowing the weight of residue and the sample weight taken for analysis, the weight in grams of the residue so can be calculated by knowing the formula and then the percentage calculations are made.

8.4 Apparatus Used in Gravimetric Analysis (Fig. 8.2)

(1) Beaker: It is a container having beak like structure and is used for preparation of solution, heating, precipitation and digestion. A borosil beaker is used as it can withstand with frequent heating and cooling. Beakers of different capacities, e.g., 50 ml, 100 ml, 500 ml and 1000 ml are available in market.

Precautions

(i) It should not be directly heated over the burner; rather a **wire gauge** should be used with asbestos sheet on lower side.

(ii) Always cover the beakers with watch glass to keep it dust free.

(2) Watch glass: Watch glass is used for covering the beaker while heating and keeping it dust free.

(3) Glass Rod: Glass rod is used to detach the particles of the precipitates, sticked on the walls of the beaker during filtrations. When the glass rod is taken out from the solution it must not be kept on the table; otherwise some part of the solutions could be decreased. It must be washed in the solution with the help of a washing solution in wash bottle.

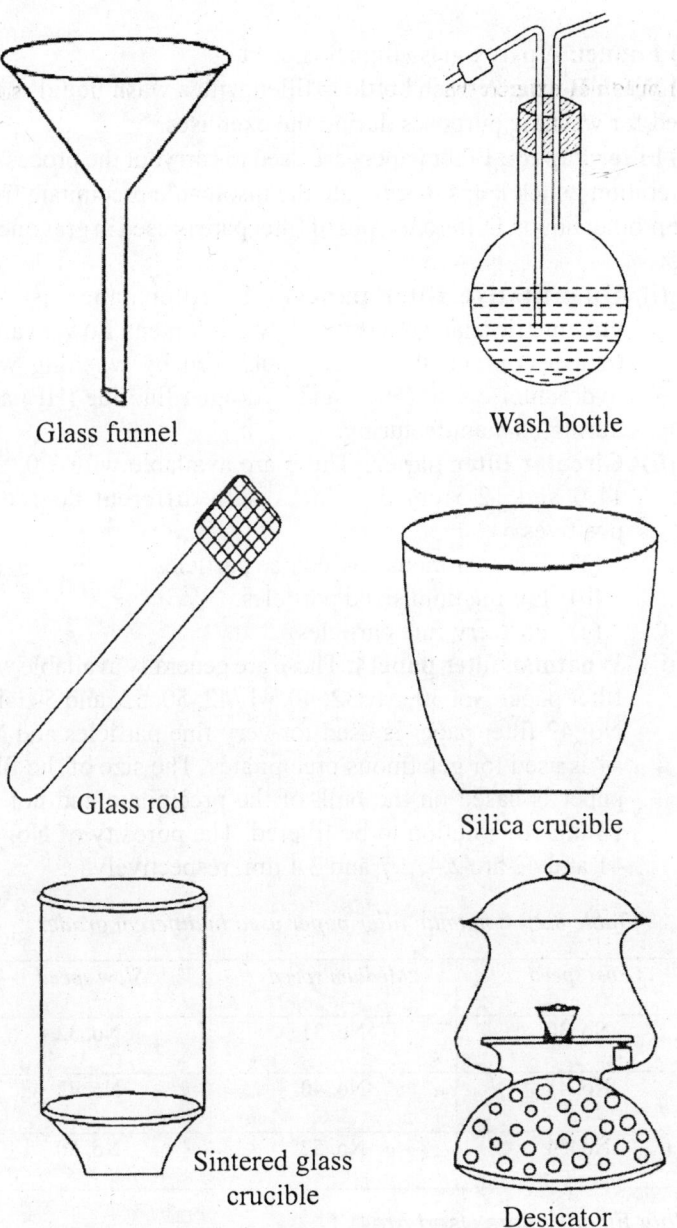

Glass funnel

Wash bottle

Glass rod

Silica crucible

Sintered glass crucible

Desicator

Fig. 8.2: Apparatus used in gravimetric analysis

(4) Funnel: A pyrex glass funnel is used.

(5) Wash Bottle: A wash bottle is filled with a wash liquid and is used for washing purposes during the exercises.

(6) Filter Papers: Filter papers are used to carryout the process of filteration which helps to separate the insoluable precipitate from the mother liquor. Different types of filter papers used in gravimetry are:

    (i) Quantitative filter paper: The filter paper used in gravimetric analysis has very low ash content. Lower values of ash content are usually achieved by washing with hydrochloric acid (HCl) and hydrogen fluoride (HF) acid during its manufacturing.

   (ii) Circular filter paper: These are available with 7.0, 9.0, 11.0 and 12.5 cm diameters with different degree of positives as:

       (a) For gelatinous and coarse particles

       (b) For medium sized particles

       (c) For very fine particles

  (iii) Whatman filter papers: These are generally available with filter paper No. 30, 31, 32, 40, 41, 42, 50, 52, and 54. The No. 42 filter paper is used for very fine particles and No. 41 is used for gelatinous precipitates. The size of the filter paper is based on the bulk of the precipitate and not the volume of solution to be filtered. The porosity of No. 40, 41 and 42 are 2.4, 2.7 and 3.1 µm, respectively.

Table 8.2: Whatman filter paper used in different grades

Fast speed	Medium speed	Slow speed
No. 30	No. 31	No. 32
No. 41	No. 40	No. 42
No. 54	No. 52	No. 50

Other Filter Papers Used Are:

- Schleicher and Schull (S and S)
- I green filter paper (I. G.)

Precautions:

(i) The filter paper used for gravimetry should not exceed the ash limit beyond 0.0001 g if its diameter is 11 cm.

(ii) If the ash content exceeds the value, it should be deducted from the weight of ignited residue.

(7) Crucible: A crucible is a cup shaped piece of laboratory equipment used to contain chemical compounds heating them to a very high temperature. The receptacle is usually made of porcelain or an inert material. The crucible should be thoroughly cleaned, ignited and dried before use. It is of two types viz:

(i) Silica crucible: The procedure of cleaning, igniting and drying of silica crucible is followed by heating with silver nitrate (HNO_3) and washing with water (H_2O). The crucible is scrubbed with moist sand and washed again with distilled water (H_2O). It is further dried with filter paper and heated in a non-luminous low flame. Slowly flame is increased and crushes ignited red to it least for five minutes. Crucible should be handled with tongs and kept in desicator for drying.

(ii) Sintered glass crucible: This type of crucible is useful for the precipitates which need no ignition and are dried by heating below 150°C. Grade No:3 is used for the precipitates of medium size as silver chloride ($AgCl$) while using sintered glass crucible, not more the 3/4 [th] of its volume should be filled with the liquid.

Advantages Over Silica Crucible

(a) Easier to clean and use.

(b) Resistant to most of chemicals.

(c) Can be heated to high temperatures.

Constant Weight of Crucible

The crucible for an elementary gravimetric work is usually made up of either protein (heat proof) or fused silica glass. The constant weight of crucible is obtained by following steps:

(i) The crucible is always placed in a desicator. It is taken out of the desicator with the help of a pair of clean tongs. The crucible is never placed on the naked table but always on a clay-pipe triangle with its legs in a standing position.

(ii) The crucible is heated strongly to red hot for 10-15 minutes with the help of a non-luminous flame. The flame is now removed and the crucible is allowed to cool to room temperature and then only transfer to desicator.

(iii) The crucible is allowed to remain inside the desicator for about 15 minutes and then it is weighed accurately up to four decimal digits/places on a chemical balance using a rider. Note down the weight.

(iv) The process of heating, cooking and weighing in the above manner is repeated, until last two consecutive readings of weight obtained are concordant. This is the constant weight of the crucible.

(v) The observations is recorded which is as follows:

Weight of the crucible $=$ (i) ... g
$=$ (ii) ... g
$=$ (iii) ... g

Constant weight of the crucible $=$ Average weight of above three readings in grams.

(8) Desicator: It is used for allowing the hot crucible to cool in a moisture free atmosphere.

Precautions

(i) While expressing the desicator, its cover should not be lifted up, rather it must be slided on it greased rim.

(ii) The cover must be kept on the table with the greased surface upwards.

(iii) Red hot crucible should never be placed directly in the desicator, first allow it to cool.

8.5 Gravimetric Precipitation

(A) Precipitate: It is a whitish curdy flake like floccules formed in the solution due to addition precipitating agents, e.g., silver nitrate ($AgNO_3$) or ammonium thiocyanate (NH_4SCN) or potassium thiocyanate ($KSCN$). Precipitate is obtained by adding suitable precipitating agent or reagent in excess from outside to given solution.

Precipitate are of two types:

Colloidal	Crystalline
(i) Particle range: 10-2000Å	(i) Size greater than 2000Å
(ii) Cannot be retained by ordinary filter paper because of smaller size	(ii) they are pure and easily filtered

Precipitation can be increased by heating, stirring and adding an electrolyte in the medium.

Characteristics of Precipitate:

(i) It must be highly insoluble.

(ii) The precipitate should be filterable.

(iii) It should be of high purity.

Saturated solution: If a solute is added to a solvent with a continuous stirring, firstly solute dissolves and a stage will come when the added solute will not dissolve any more but settles down at the bottom of the container. As this stage solution is called saturated solution. In saturated solution the dissolved substance is in equilibrium with undissolved substances present at the bottom of the container.

Supersaturated solutions: A supersaturated solution is an unstable solution that contains a higher solute concentration. As compared to saturated solution the supersaturated solution contains greater amount of dissolved substances that undissolved substances. This is achieved by heating the saturated solution. The state of super saturation is unstable and exists only for a short period of time.

Mechanism of Precipitate

The formation of the precipitate involves two stages:

(1) Nucleation

It is a process in which a minimum number of atoms, ions or molecules join together to give stable solids. It also involves the formation of nucleus and is further classified into two types as:

(i) **Spontaneous:** Sometimes it is possible in supersaturated solution, ions will join together to form nucleus. It is called spontaneous nucleation and will occur its own.

(ii) **Induced:** If a small crystal of solute is added to the supersaturated solution, it will act as a nucleus for growth of a crystal. It is called induced nucleation and requires a seed particle to get things started.

(2) Crystal Growth

It is achieved after nucleation. It is observed in two cases:

(i) Diffusion of ions to the surface of growing crystal.

(ii) Deposition of these diffused ions on crystal surface.

Once the nucleation site is formed the other ions are attracted to the site and will result in the formation of large, filterable particles.

Contamination of Precipitate

Despite of all precautions during precipitation, the unwanted ions are carried down with the precipitate from solutions. This is called contamination of precipitate. The contamination may be due to several reasons, but mainly it is of two types;

(1) Co-precipitation (Precipitating Together)

If sulphuric acid (H_2SO_4) is added to the solution of containing a mixture of barium chloride ($BaCl_2$) and ferric chloride ($FeCl_3$), we would expect only barium sulphate ($BaSO_4$) to be precipitated, since the other salt formed is ferrous sulphate [$Fe_2(SO_4)_3$] and is soluble in water (H_2O). However, in reality the salt is partially precipitated and this can be seen if the precipitate is filtered off, washed and ignited. The residue is not white [(the color of barium sulphate ($BaSO_4$)] but is colored brownish by ferric oxide which is formed by the decomposition of $Fe_2(SO_4)_3$ on heating:

$$Fe_2(SO_4)_3 \xrightarrow{\Delta} Fe_2O_3 + \uparrow 3SO_3$$

Ferrous sulphate   Ferric oxide
(brownish)

Therefore, precipitation of any soluble or extraneous substance along with the precipitate is called as co-precipitation. The co-precipitation literally means 'precipitating together'. Due to co-precipitation some soluble impurity may get incorporated along with into the precipitate. Therefore, co-precipitation is one of the most important source of error is gravimetric analysis or determination because the weighed form containing co-precipitated impurities in no longer pure substance. Hence, exact calculation of the pure substance amount of the element being to be determined is impossible. The analysis performing gravimetric determination must consistently take steps to diminish co-precipitation of impurities and the precipitant itself. The phenomenon used for the removal of soluble substance from the solution by the precipitate are:

   (i) Surface adsorption/adsorption co-precipitation.

  (ii) Mixed crystal formation/isomorphous co-precipitation.

 (iii) Occlusion.

 (iv) Mechanical occlusion.

The Co-Precipitation Occurs When

  (a) Co-precipitated material and host material have the same crystal structure.

  (b) Like host material the co-precipitated ion must not be very soluble, because less soluble things forms solid solutions to a greater extent than more soluble once i.e. solubility product is in equilibrium to host material.

(i) Adsorption Co-Precipitation

In this type of co-precipitation, the ion impurity is adsorbed on the surface of freshly formed primary precipitate during its formation from the solution.

$$BaCl_2 \ + \ Na_2SO_4 \ \longrightarrow \ BaSO_4\downarrow \ + \ 2\,NaCl$$

| Barium chloride | Sodium sulphate | Barium sulphate | Sodium chloride |

The Ba^{+2} ions are adsorbed on the precipitate of barium sulphate ($BaSO_4$) because the multi charged ion has greater affinity to adsorb on a single charged ion.

(ii) Isomorphous co-precipitation: (Formation of mixed-crystals)

Substances are said to be isomorphous if they crystallize with the formation of a joint crystal lattice, so called mixed crystals are formed in the process. Hence, the isomorphism exists between precipitate with the co- precipitate impurity. If a mixture of the colorless potash alum $KAl(SO_4)_2$. $12H_2O$ and the deep violet chrome alum $KCr(SO_4)_2$. $12 H_2O$ is dissolved in water (H_2O) and left to crystallize, mixed crystals are formed. Isomorphous substances have formulae of the same type.

(iii) Occlusion

It is trapping of ionic impurities within the crystal and formation of solid solution by both. Less soluble ions are occluded most, e.g., nitrate occluded on $BaSO_4$. The co-precipitated impurities are within the precipitate particle.

(iv) Mechanical Entrapment

Crystals grown under practical condition is hardly ever 'ideal', i.e., do not form quite regular crystal lattices. They contain minute cracks and cavities filled with the mother liquid. Very small crystal are apt to aggregate, entertaining the mother liquor the faster crystallization occurs, the more of such impurities will be entertained because on fast crystallization. The ions do not have time, as it were, to form a regular crystal lattice. This type of co-precipitation is known as *mechanical occlusion*.

(2) Post Precipitation (After Precipitation)

The precipitation of the impurity on the surface of the primary precipitate after its formation is called post precipitation. In this process a gradual deposition of impurity occurs at the surface of precipitate, when the solution and precipitate are left is contact for longer hours. For example Ca^{2+} can be precipitated as oxalate from the solution containing both calcium and magnesium, but if the precipitate is allowed to stand for considerable length of time, magnesium-oxalate is post-precipitated on the surface of calcium-oxalate. The phenomenon of post precipitation is of great importance in the quantitative estimation of metal ion with H_2S

gas, e.g., zinc is not precipitated with H_2S gas in weakly acidic solution, but if H_2S gas is passed and the solution is allowed to stand for a long time, ZnS is post precipitated along with the sulphide of other metal ions. It occurs whether contaminant or impurity causing the post-precipitation is added to liquid after the precipitate forms. Post precipitation depends upon following factors;

(i) It increases with time.

(ii) It increases at higher temperature.

In post-precipitation, the impurity remains in supersaturated conditions on mother liquor and the primary precipitate provided nuclei for the deposition of impurity.

Post precipitation can be minimized by;

(a) Eliminating the process of digestion.

(b) Addition of immiscible liquid after formation of precipitate, and

(c) Decreasing material agitation of solutions.

Table 8.3: *Difference between co-precipitation and post precipitation*

° Co-precipitation	Post precipitation
The precipitation of any soluble or extraneous substance along with the precipitate	The precipitation of the impurity on the surface of the primary precipitate after its formation
It is caused when there is contamination of precipitate with soluble impurities	It is caused when the precipitate is left for longer time with mother liquor (digestion)
It has greater extent of contamination	It has less content of contamination
It increase with agitation of solution	It decreases with agitation of solution

(B) Digestion of Precipitate

Digestion is the process in which the precipitate is allowed to stand with mother liquor for about 10-12 hours at room temperature or warming the precipitate for sometime in contact with the solution from which it was precipitate (mother liquor). No washing is done if the precipitate is gelatinous or if there is a possibility of post-precipitation.

The processes of digestion results in the formation of bigger particles of the precipitate. The precipitates are easily filterable, as more reactive finer particle of the precipitate and also those which are present at the sharp edges (active step) tend to dissolve in the mother liquor. They redeposit on the larger particles that are easily to filter. Here the occluded impurities get an opportunity to escape in the solution, hence co-precipitation is minimized. The process of digestion makes precipitate:

(i)   Pure.

(ii)   Easily filterable than initial precipitate.

(iii)   Of greater particle size.

Peptization: Some freshly precipitated substances such as silver chloride (AgCl), ferric hydroxide and aluminum hydroxide can be readily converted into colloidal solution by the addition of a small amount of a strong electrolyte. Thus on adding a small amount of a dilute solution of ferric chloride ($FeCl_3$ $6H_2O$) to the freshly precipitated ferric hydroxide [$Fe(OH)_3$], a reddish brown solution of ferric hydroxide is formed. Similarly if to a precipitate of stannic oxide, a small amount of dilute HCl is added, a stable solution of stannic oxide results. The process of transferring back to a precipitate into colloidal state is called *peptization*.

A substance like ferric chloride ($FeCl_3.6H_2O$) or dilute hydrochloric acid (HCl) is called a peptizing agent. The Fe^{3+} ions are adsorbed on particles of Fe $(OH)_3$ precipitate, whereby positive charge comes on their surface.

(C) Filtration of precipitate: During filtration, the level of liquid in the funnel should not be allowed to rinse above 1 cm from the edge of the paper. If the precipitate is sticking to the sides of the beaker, the same is removed with the help of glass rod and the wash liquid. The solution is again decanted off as before and the washed precipitation is then carefully transferred into the filter paper with the help of glass rod and washed again (Fig. 8.2). The commonly used filter paper for the filtration of precipitate is Whatman filter paper no. 42 with porosity of 3.1 μm.

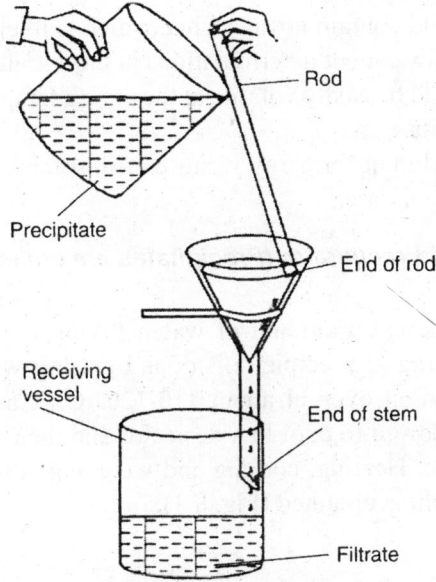

Fig. 8.2: *Filteration of precipitate*

Precautions During Filtration of Precipitate

1. It should be carried by decantation.
2. No drop of liquid should be wasted during filtration.
3. No precipitate should be left behind in the beaker.
4. Filter paper must be struck properly on the walls of the funnel.

(D) Washing in Gravimetric Analysis

Most precipitates are produced in the presence of one or more soluble compounds. Since the soluble compounds are frequently non-volatile at the drying temperature of the precipitate, it is necessary to wash the precipitate to remove impurities as completely as possible. The ideal washing solution should comply following conditions:

(i) It should have not solvent action on the precipitate, but dissolve foreign substance easily.

(ii) It should have no dispersive action on a precipitate.

(iii) It should contain no substance which is likely to interfere with subsequent determinations in the filtrate.

(iv) It should be easily volatile at the drying temperature of the precipitate.

(v) It should not form any volatile or in soluble product with the precipitate.

(E) Drying of Precipitate: (Precipitates are collected on filter paper)

To remove the extra amount of water, drying is required after washing. Drying of precipitate is done by using Whatman filter paper dried in an oven at about 110-120° C. After drying, the crucible is allowed to cool in a desicator and then weighed with the precipitate. Heating, cooling and weighing is repeated till a constant weight is obtained (Fig. 8.3).

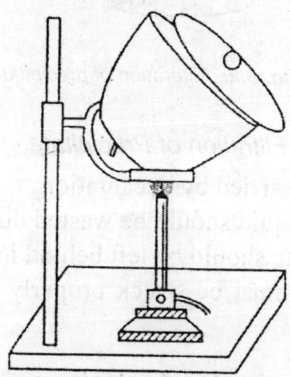

Fig.8.3: Drying of precipitate

(F) Ignition of Precipitate

The Ignition of the precipitate can be described under following two headings:

1. Ignition and the incarnation of filter paper

The filter paper having precipitate is taken out of the funnel carefully and opened in such a way that the fingers do not touch the precipitate. Alternatively, the precipitate may also be collected over a clean and dry glazed paper. Take the help of the feather or camel brush to collect the fine particles of the precipitate. Now cover the precipitate with a funnel and keep it safe. Fold the filter paper several times so that it looks like a long small cone. Catch the top side of the cone with a pair of tongs by one hand and ignite the cone by means of a flame by the burner in other hand horizontally (Fig. 8.4). Collect the ash in a previously weighed crucible placed on a glazed paper. The crucible is then heated strongly to brush off all the carbon to a white ash (may not be white, e.g.; in case of Fe and Cu).

2. Treatment of the Ash

During ignition the small fraction of the precipitate may get reduced by the carbon of the paper into a compound (or metal) altogether different from the compound in which determination is sought. The ash is treated with suitable regents to get back the form (compound) in which it is finally to be weighed. The step is called the **ash treatment** (Fig. 8.4).

Ignition of precipitate is done in constantly weighed silica crucible. The filter paper containing the precipitate by keeping it in a tongue and its ash is collected in the crucible placed on a glazed paper. When all the ash has been collected in the crucible, it is now subjected to red-heat.

(G) Weighing of Precipitate

Crucible containing the precipitate is weighed and the weight of the precipitate may be obtained as:

   (i) Weight of empty crucible $= x$ grams

  (ii) Weight of crucible + precipitate $= y$ grams

 (iii) Weight of precipitate $= (y - x) = z$ grams

8.6 Thermogravimetric Method of Analysis

Thermogravimetry is a technique in which change in weight of a substance is recorded as a function of temperature. The curves which are used to determine the temperature at which the precipitate may be dried or ignited to the required chemical form are called **thermogravimetric curves.**

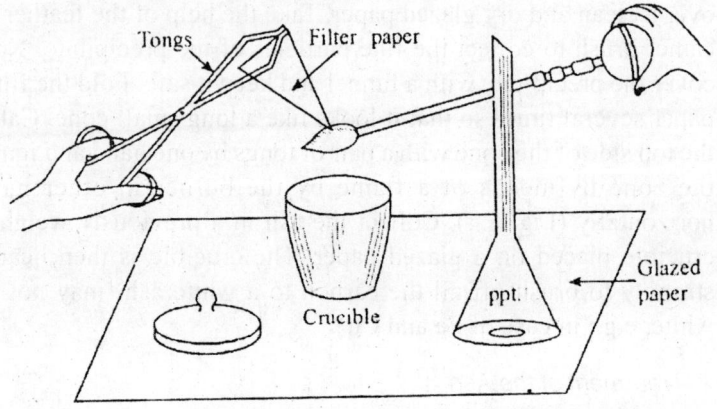

Fig. 8.4: Ash treatment

The study and results of thermogravimetric analysis (TGA) may be represented in two ways.

1. As a thermogravimetric (TG) curve, in which the weight change is recorded as a function of temperature.
2. As a derivative thermogravimetric (DTG) curve where the first derivative of the TG curve is plotted with respect to either temperature.

Since TG curve is quantitative, calculations on compound stoichiometry can be made at any given temperature. In the rate of change of weight with time dw/dt is plotted against temperature, a derivative thermogravimetric (DTG) curve is obtained (Fig. 8.5).

In the DTG curve when there is no weight loss then dw/dt = 0. The peak on the derivative curve corresponds to a maximum slope on the TG curve. When dw/dt is minimum but not zero, there is an inflection, i.e., changing of slope on a TG curve.

Advantages the thermogravimetric analysis

1. It is precise and accurate when using modern analytical balances.
2. Possible sources of error are readily checked since filtrates can be checked for completeness of precipitation and precipitates may be examined for the presence of impurities.
3. It is an absolute method, i.e., it involves direct measurement without any form of calibrations being required.

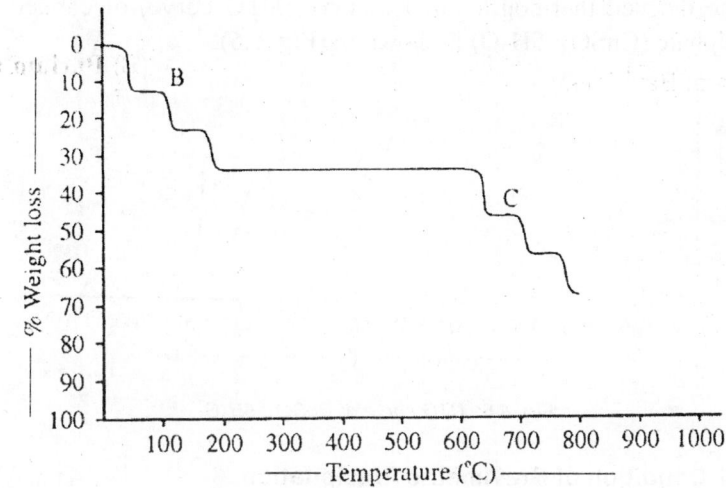

Fig.8.5: *Thermogravimetric (TG) curve.*

4. Determination can be carried out with relatively inexpensive apparatus: the most expensive items are a muffle furnace and sometimes platinum crucible.
5. It is possible to achieve high level of accuracy and separatibility of results with 0.3-0.5%.

Applications

(i) In determinations of purity and thermal stability of primary and secondary standard.
(ii) For the investigation of correct drying temperature
(iii) For the determination of composition of complex mixtures.
(iv) Analysis of standards used for the testing and/or calibrations of instrumental techniques.
(v) Analysis requiring high accuracy.

Thermal decomposition of $CuSO_4.5H_2O$		*Approx tempt.*
1. $CuSO_4. 5H_2O$	$CuSO_4.H_2O$	90–150°C
2. $CuSO_4. H_2O$	$CuSO_4$	200–275°C
3. $CuSO_4$	$CuO + SO_2 + \frac{1}{2} O_2$	700–900°C
4. $2CuO$	$Cu_2O + \frac{1}{2} O_2$	1000–1100 °C

The derived thermogravimetric curve (DTG curve) of copper sulphate ($CuSO_4 . 5H_2O$) is shown in (Fig. 8.6).

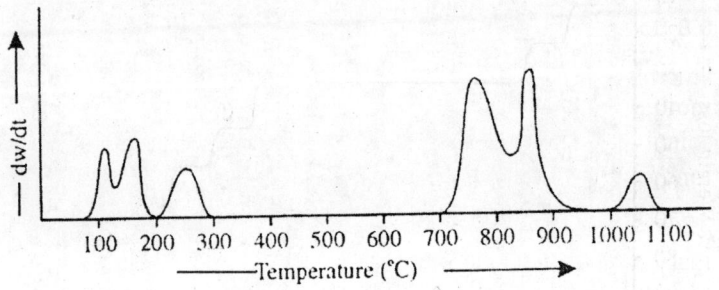

Fig. 8.6: *DTG curve of $CuSO_4 . 5H_2O$*

8.7 Condition of Gravimetric Precipitation

In gravimetric analysis, precipitation is carried out under such experimental conditions that are rapid and complete. Condition must be such which may yield large sized particle which do not pass through the filtering medium and their must be minimum contamination of the precipitate.

   (i) Concentration of reagent: The precipitation should be carried in dilute solution.

  (ii) Rate of addition of reagent: A dilute solution of the precipitating reagent should be added slowly with constant stirring of the solution. It helps in the growth of large crystals by keeping the degree of supersaturation small.

 (iii) Temperature of solution: Precipitation in hot solution helps in coagulation and also causes better growth of crystals of the precipitates. Further it checks post precipitation.

  (iv) Quantity of reagent: A slight excess of reagent (large excess is avoided) is required to ensure complete precipitation.

   (v) Digestion of precipitate: It helps in bigger size of crystals and is carried in steam bath. This process is not important in case of amorphous or gelatinous precipitates and helps in decreasing the co-precipitation.

(vi) pH of the solution: Precipitation of ca-oxalate is carried out is a mildly acidic solution followed by the addition of aqueous ammonia.

8.8 Organic Precipitants

Organic precipitants or reagent are used for the precipitation of inorganic reagents and precipitation is done in hot and dilute solutions. These are used for the separation of one or more inorganic ions from mixtures by interacting with them.

Organic precipitants are usually of high molecular weight so that small amount of ions will yield relatively large amount of precipitate. These precipitates are sparingly soluble (30 to 100 parts of solvent required to dissolve 1 part of solute) and usually colored.

Advantages of Organic Precipitants

1. They form characteristics color with the ions to be detected.

2. The precipitate produced with the help of organic reagents have low affinity for water (H_2O), thus can be easily dried at low temperature without decomposition.

3. They are very sensitive and are capable of detecting an extremely small amount of substances, e.g., as below as 10 mg.

4. They are specific in nature and can be used for the detection of single type of ion in a complex mixture.

5. They form the insoluble precipitate or chelate (disodium EDTA) of high molecular weight.

Important Organic Precipitates Are

1. Dimethyl glyoxime.

$$CH_3 - C = NOH$$
$$\qquad\quad |$$
$$CH_3 - C = NOH$$

Uses: (1) Determination of nickel (Ni) in steel.

(2) Detection of bismuth (Bi) and palladium (Pd)

$$2 \begin{array}{c} CH_3-C=NOH \\ | \\ CH_3-C=NOH \end{array} + NiCl_2 + 2NH_4OH \rightarrow \begin{array}{c} OH \cdots O \\ | \quad \uparrow \\ CH_3-C=N \quad N=C-CH_3 \\ | \quad Ni \quad | \\ CH_3-C=N \quad N=C-CH_3 \\ \downarrow \quad | \\ O \quad OH \end{array}$$

$$+ 2NH_4Cl + 2H_2O$$

It gives a bright red precipitate with Na^+ salt solution in alkaline medium. The precipitate or complex is weighed after drying at 110-120°C.

2. 1-Nitroso-2-naphthol (α-nitroso-β-naphthol)

(red brown precipitate)

Uses: (1) For the precipitation of many metallic ions, e.g., Fe, Cl and Co.

(2) The reagent don't react with Ni. It can be used for the separation of Ni from cobalt.

3. Cupferon: It gives precipitates with Fe^{3+}, Ti^{4+} and Ce^{3+}. It is specific precipitating agent for potassium acid ammonium ions.

$$C_6H_5N (NO) ONH_4 + FeCl_3 \rightarrow [C_6H_5N (NO) O]_3 Fe + 3NH_4Cl$$
nitrosophenyl hydroxyl amine

Some **inorganic** precipitating agents are given as: ammonia $[NH_3(aq)]$, hydrogen sulphide (H_2S), sulphuric acid (H_2SO_4), silver nitrate $(AgNO_3)$, ammonium thiocyanate (NH_4SCN), ammonium chloride (NH_4Cl), barium chloride $(BaCl_2)$, magnesium chloride $(MgCl_2)$ and sodium bicarbonate $(NaHCO_3)$.

8.9 Specific Example of Gravimetric Analysis

(A); Aluminium as Al₂O₃ (Aluminium Oxide)

Principle: Aluminium is precipitated as aluminium hydrous oxide, $Al_2O_3 \cdot xH_2O$ by the addition of aqueous ammonia as ammonium hydroxide (NH_4OH) to an aluminum salt solution. A white gelatinous precipitate of aluminium hydroxide is obtained which is ignited and weighed as aluminium oxide (Al_2O_3).

$$Al_2(SO_4)_3 + 6\,NH_4OH \longrightarrow 2\,Al\,(OH)_3^- + 3\,(NH_4)_2\,SO_4$$
Aluminium sulphate   Aluminium hydroxide

$$2Al\,(OH)_3 \longrightarrow Al_2O_3 + 3\,H_2O$$
Aluminium oxide

The precipitation is usually carried out in the presence of NH_4Cl (added solid) and a few drops of methyl red indicator (0.2% alcoholic solution).

Procedure: Pipette out 25 ml of the given solution into 500 ml beaker. Add 100 ml of distilled water, 5 g of ammonium chloride (NH_4Cl) and 0.3 ml of methyl red solution. Dissolve the salt and heat the resulting solution to boiling. To this hot solution, add 50% ammonia (NH_3) solution drop wise with constant stirring until the solution gets yellow color. Boil the solution again for 1-2 min and allow the precipitate to settle down. Test the supernatant liquid for complete precipitation. Now filter the precipitate by decantation method through Whatman filter paper no. 42. Wash the precipitate 3-4 times with hot water and dry it by placing the funnel in an oven. After drying transfer the filter paper containing the precipitate to the pre-constantly weighed crucible and ignite it till all the carbonaceous matter is not burnt off. Now cool the crucible and add one drop each of conc. hydrochloric acid (HCl) and conc. sulphuric acid (Ash treatment). Cool the crucible by placing it in a desicator and weigh it. Repeat the process of heating, igniting, cooling and weighing till the constant weight is obtained.

Calculations/Gravimetric factor: After the precipitation let the weight of the aluminium dioxide (Al_2O_3) precipitate be x grams.

$$Al_2O_3 = 2\,Al = K_2SO_4 \cdot H_2(SO_4)_2 \cdot 24\,H_2O$$
$$101.94 \quad 53.94 \quad 948.85$$
$$101.94 \text{ g of } Al_2O_3 \text{ contains} = 53.94 \text{ g of } Al$$

$$\therefore x \text{ grams of } Al_2O_3 \text{ contains} = \frac{53.94 \times x}{101.94} \text{ g of } Al$$

Precautions:

1. Precipitation should be carried out in a dilute hot solution.
2. Concentration of NH_3 ions must not exceed certain limits because

the solubility of hydrated Al_2O_3 increases in an excess of ammonia (NH_3).

(B) Barium as $BaSO_4$: (Barium sulphate)

Principle: When dilute sulphuric acid (H_2SO_4) is added to a dilute solution of barium chloride $(BaCl_2)$, a white precipitate of barium sulphate $(BaSO_4)$ is formed.

$$BaCl_2 + H_2SO_4 \rightarrow BaSO_4 + 2HCl$$

A white gelatinous precipitate is obtained which is filtered, washed, dried, ignited and weighed as barium sulphate $(BaSO_4)$.

Reagents Used

1. Barium chloride $(BaCl_2)$ solution (12.57 g in 1000 ml of distilled water).
2. Precipitating agent (3 ml of conc. H_2SO_4 in 100 ml of D.W).
3. Wash solution (Hot distilled water).

Procedure: Pipette out 25 ml of the given solution of barium chloride $(BaCl_2)$ into 500 ml beaker. Add 0.5 ml of concentrated sulphuric acid (H_2SO_4) and 100 ml of distilled water. Heat the resulting solution to boiling. To this hot solution, add dilute sulphuric acid (H_2SO_4) solution drop wise with constant stirring until the precipitation is not complete. Allow the precipitate to settle down and test the supernatant liquid for complete precipitation. Now filter the precipitate by decantation method through Whatman filter paper no.42. Wash the precipitate 3-4 times by decantation with hot water. Dry the precipitate by placing the funnel in an oven. After drying transfer the filter paper containing the precipitate to the pre-constantly weighed crucible and ignite it till all the carbonaceous matter is not burnt off. Now cool the crucible and add one drop each of conc. hydrochloric acid HCl and conc. sulphuric acid $[H_2SO_4]$ (Ash treatment). Cool the crucible by placing it in a desicator and weigh it. Repeat the process of heating, igniting, cooling and weighing till the constant weight is obtained.

Calculations/Gravimetric factor

Let the constant weight of barium sulphate $(BaSO_4)$ precipitate be x grams.

$$BaSO_4 \equiv Ba$$

$$233.42 \equiv 137.36$$

233.42 g of $BaSO_4$ contains = 137.36 g of Ba^{2+} ions.

$\therefore$ x grams of $BaSO_4$ contains = $\dfrac{137.36 \text{ g}}{233.42}$ g × x g. of Ba^{2+} ions.

Precautions

1. Precipitation should be carried out in a dilute hot solution

2. Precipitation should be carried out in the presence of 0.05 N conc. HCl which helps to increase the size of the precipitate particles.

EXERCISES

---

1. What is gravimetric analysis? Discuss in detail principle and theory involved.

2. Write a note on co-precipitation and post-precipitation in gravimetry.

3. Give characteristics of the apparatus used in gravimetric analysis.

4. Write a note on filtration and drying in gravimetric analysis.

5. How will you get constant weight of crucible? Estimate aluminium (Al) as aluminium oxide (Al_2O_3).

6. Discuss ignition, peptization, digestion and organic precipitants in gravimetry.

7. What are the different types of filter papers used in gravimetric analysis?

8. Write a note on thermogravimetry. What are its advantages?

9. Give characteristics of the washing solution in gravimetric analysis?

10. Name and explain in detail the common apparatus used in gravimetric analysis.

11. What are saturated and supersaturated solutions?

12. What is the difference between gravimetric and volumetric analysis?

13. What is the purpose of the washing of the precipitate?

14. What type of the filter papers are used for filtration?

15. Discuss the precautions to be taken in filtration, washing, incineration and digestion of the precipitate.

16. Explain the thermal decomposition of the copper sulphate pentahydrate.

17. What do understand by organic precipitants?

18. Illustrate your discussion by examples of gravimetric estimation of aluminum as aluminum oxide?

19. Discuss solubility product with reference to the gravimetry.

20. Estimate barium (Ba) as Barium sulphate ($BaSO_4$).

Appendix

Table A.1: Elements-symbols, Atomic numbers and their Atomic weights

Name(Symbol)	Atomic number	Atomic weight
Actinium (Ac)	89	227
Aluminium (Al)	13	27
Americium (Am)	95	243
Antimony (Sb)	51	121
Argon (Ar)	18	40
Arsenic (As)	33	75
Astatine (At)	85	210
Barium (Ba)	56	137
Berkelium (Bk)	97	247
Beryllium (Be)	4	9
Bismuth (Bi)	83	209
Boron (B)	5	11
Bromine (Br)	35	80
Cadmium (Cd)	48	112
Calcium (Ca)	20	40
Californium (Cf)	98	251
Carbon (C)	6	12
Cerium (Ce)	58	140
Cesium (Cs)	55	133

Contd.

Chlorine (Cl)	17	35.45
Chromium (Cr)	24	52
Cobalt (Co)	27	59
Copper (Cu)	29	63.5
Curium (Cm)	96	246
Dysprosium (Dy)	66	163
Einsteinium (Es)	99	252
Erbium (Er)	68	167
Europium (Eu)	63	152
Fermium (Fm)	100	257
Fluorine (F)	9	19
Francium (Fr)	87	223
Gadolinium (Gd)	64	157
Gallium (Ga)	31	69
Germanium (Ge)	32	72.6
Gold (Au)	79	197
Hafnium (Hf)	72	178.4
Helium (He)	2	4.002
Holmium (Ho)	67	165
Hydrogen (H)	1	1.007
Indium (In)	49	115
Iodine (I)	53	126.9
Iridium (Ir)	77	192.2
Iron (Fe)	26	55.8
Krypton (Kr)	36	83
Lanthanum (La)	57	139
Lawrencium (Lr)	103	262
Lead (Pb)	82	207
Lithium (Li)	3	6.9
Lutetium (Lu)	71	175
Magnesium (Mg)	12	24.3
Manganese (Mn)	25	54.9

Contd.

Mendelevium (Md)	101	258
Mercury (Hg)	80	200.5
Molybdenum (Mo)	42	96
Neodymium (Nd)	60	144
Neon (Ne)	10	20.1
Neptunium (Np)	93	237
Nickel (Ni)	28	58.6
Niobium (Nb)	41	93
Nitrogen (N)	7	14
Nobelium (No)	102	259
Osmium (Os)	76	190
Oxygen (O)	8	15.9
Palladium (Pd)	46	106.4
Phosphorus (P)	15	30.9
Platinum (Pt)	78	195
Plutonium (Pu)	84	209
Potassium (K)	19	39
Praseodymium (Pr)	59	140.9
Promethium (Pm)	61	145
Protactinium (Pa)	91	231
Radium (Ra)	88	226
Radon (Rn)	86	222
Rhenium (Re)	75	186
Rubidium (Rb)	37	85.4
Ruthenium (Ru)	44	101
Samarium (Sm)	62	150
Scandium (Sc)	21	45
Selenium (Se)	34	78.9
Silicon (Si)	14	28
Silver (Ag)	47	106.9
Sodium (Na)	11	23
Sulfur (S)	16	32

Contd.

Tantalum (Ta)	73	180
Technetium (Tc)	43	98
Tellurium (Te)	52	127.6
Terbium (Tb)	65	159
Thallium (Tl)	81	204
Thorium (Th)	90	232
Thulium (Tm)	69	168
Tin (Sn)	50	118
Titanium (Ti)	22	47
Tungsten (W)	74	183
Unnilennium (Une)	109	267
Unnilhexium (Unh)	106	263
Unniloctium (Uno)	108	265
Unnilpentium (Unp)	105	262
Unnilquaderium (Unq)	104	261
Unnilseptium (Uns)	107	262
Uranium (U)	92	238
Vanadium (V)	23	51
Xenon (Xe)	54	131.2
Ytterbium (Yb)	70	173
Yttrium (Y)	39	89
Zinc (Zn)	30	65.3
Zirconium (Zr)	40	91

Table A.2: Equivalent weight of some compounds

Compound (formula)	Molecular weight	Acidity/Basicity/ loss or gain of electron	Equivalent weight
Hydrochloric acid (HCl)	36.46	1	36.46
Nitric acid (HNO$_3$)	63.01	1	63.01
Sulphuric acid (H$_2$SO$_4$)	98.07	2	49.03
Acetic acid (CH$_3$COOH)	60.05	1	60.05
Boric acid (H$_3$BO$_3$)	61.83	3	20.16
Sodium hydroxide (NaOH)	40.0	1	40.00
Potassium hydroxide (KOH)	56.11	1	56.11
Sodium carbonate (Na$_2$CO$_3$)	105.99	2	53.00
Sodium bicarbonate (NaHCO$_3$)	84.01	1	84.01
Potassium carbonate (K$_2$CO$_3$)	138.21	2	69.10
Potassium permanganate (KMmO$_4$)	158.03	5	31.60

Contd.

Potassium dichromate ($K_2Cr_2O_7$)	294.18	6	49.03
Iodine (I_2)	253.8	2	126.90
Oxalic acid anhydrous $(COOH)_2$	90.0	2	45.00
Oxalic acid dihydrate $(COOH)_2 \cdot 2H_2O$	126.07	2	63.03
Sodium thiosulphate $Na_2S_2O_3 \cdot 5H_2O$	248.17	1	248.17

Table A.3: Primary and secondary standards- equivalent weight, preparation and strength

Reagents	Equivalent weight (EW)	Preparation	Strength
Hydrochloric acid(HCl)	36.5	Dissolve 8.5 ml of concentrated HCl in 1000 ml of water	0.1 N
Ammonium thiocyanate (NH_4SCN)	76.10	Dissolve 7.610 g of NH_4SCN in 1000 ml of water	0.1 N
Copper sulphate ($CuSO_4$. $5H_2O$)	249.71	Dissolve 24.9 g of $CuSO_4$. $5H_2O$ in 1000 ml of water	0.1 N
Oxalic acid ($H_2C_2O_4$. $2H_2O$)	63.04	Dissolve 6.304 g of $H_2C_2O_4.2H_2O$ in 1000 ml of water	0.1 N
Potassium dichromate ($K_2Cr_2O_7$)	49.03	Dissolve 49.03 g of $K_2Cr_2O_7$ in 1000 ml of water	1 N
Potassium permanganate ($KMnO_4$)	31.6	Dissolve 31.06 of $KMnO_4$ in 1000 ml of water	1 N
Sodium Chloride (NaCl)	58.46	Dissolve 58.46 of NaCl in 1000 ml of water	1 N
Sodium Carbonate (Na_2CO_3)	53	Dissolve 5.3 g of Na_2CO_3 in 1000 ml of water	0.1 N
Sodium Hydroxide (NaOH)	40	Dissolve 40 g of NaOH in 1000 ml of water	1 N
Iodine (I_2)	63.50	Dissolve 6.35 g of I_2 in 1000 ml of water	0.1 N

Contd.

Silver nitrate ($AgNO_3$)	169.9	Dissolve of 16.9 g $AgNO_3$ in 1000 ml of water	0.1 N
Sodium thiosulphate ($Na_2S_2O_3 \cdot 5H_2O$)	248.20	Dissolve 24.8 g of in 1000 ml of water	0.1 N
Potassium thiocyanate (KCNS)	97.16	Dissolve 9.716 g of KCNS in 1000 ml of water	0.1 N
Sulphuric acid (H_2SO_4)	49	Dissolve 28 ml of Conc. H_2SO_4 in 1000 ml of water	1 N

Indicators
Table A.4: Acid base indicators

Indicator	Transition pH range	Low pH color (Color in acidic solution)	High pH color(Color in basic
Thymol blue (1st)	1.2-2.8	Red	Yellow
Methyl yellow	2.9-4.0	Red	Yellow
Bromophenol blue	3.0-4.6	Yellow	Purple
Congo red	3.0-5.0	Blue-violet	Red
Methyl orange	3.1-4.4	Red	Yellow
Bromocresol green	3.8-5.4	Yellow	Blue-green
Methyl red	4.4-6.2	Red	Yellow
Bromocresol purple	5.2-6.8	Yellow	Purple
Bromocresol blue	6.0-7.6	Yellow	Blue
Phenol red	6.8-8.4	Yellow	Red
Neutral red	6.8-8.0	Red	Yellow
Thymol blue (2nd)	8.0-9.6	Yellow	Blue
Naptholpthalein	7.3-8.7	Colorless	Greenish-blue
Phenolphthalein	8.3-10.1	Colorless	Pink
Thymolphthalein	9.3-10.5	Colorless	Blue

Table A.5: Adsorption indicators

Indicator	Use	Experimental conditions	Color change at end - point
1. Fluorescein	Halides, e.g., I^-, Cl^-, Br^- with Ag^+.	Neutral or weakly basic solution	Yellow green-Pink
2. Tetrazine	Ag^+ with I^- or SCN-excess Ag+ on back titration, i.e., I^-.	Back titration	Colorless-Green
3. Dichloro-fluorocein	Cl^-, Br^- with Ag^+	PH range 4.4 – 7.0	Yellow green-Red

Table A.6: Redox indicators

Indicator	$E^0(V)$	Color of Ox. form	Color of Red. form
2,2'-Bipyridine	+1.33 V	Colorless	Yellow
n-Phenylan-thranilic acid	+1.08 V	Violet-red	Colorless
Diphenylamine	+0.76 V	Violet	Colorless
Sodium dipheny-lamine sulfonate	+0.84 V	Red-violet	Colorless
Diphenyl-benzidine	+0.76 V	Violet	Colorless

Table A.7: Non-aqueous indicators

Indicator	Basic	Neutral	Acidic
Crystal Violet (0.5 per cent in glacial acetic acid)	Violet	Blue-green	Yellowish-green
α-Naphtholbenzein (0.2 per cent in glacial acetic acid)	Green	Orange	Dark-green
Oracet Blue B (0.5 per cent in glacial acetic acid)	Blue or blue green	Purple	Pink
Quinaldine Red (0.1 per cent in methanol)	Magenta	—	Almost colorless

Glossary

Absolute error: Compare with relative error. The uncertainty in a measurement, expressed with appropriate units. For example, if three replicate weights for an object are 1.00 g, 1.05 g, and 0.95 g, the absolute error can be expressed as ± 0.05 g. Absolute error is also used to express inaccuracies; for example, if the "true value" is 1.11 g and the measured value is 1.00 g, the absolute error could be written as 1.00 g – 1.11 g = –0.11 g.

Accuracy: The 'accuracy' of a determination may be defined as the closeness between measured value and true or most probable value. Accuracy is the correctness of a single measurement. The accuracy of a measurement is assessed by comparing the measurement with the true or accepted value, based on evidence independent of the measurement. The closeness of an **average** to a true value is referred to as "trueness".

Acetic Acid: (CH_3COOH, $HC_2H_3O_2$) ethanoic acid; vinegar acid; methane carboxylic acid. A simple organic acid that gives vinegar its characteristic odor and flavor. Glacial acetic acid is pure acetic acid.

Acid: (Lat. acidus, sour) Compare with base. 1. A compound which releases hydrogen ions (H^+) in solution (Arrhenius). 2. A compound containing detachable hydrogen ions (Bronsted-Lowry). 3. A compound that can accept a pair of electrons from a base (Lewis).

Acidimetry titration: It is a direct or residual volumetric analysis of a base with a standard acid.

Acid anhydride: Nonmetallic oxides or organic compounds that react with water to form acids. For example, SO_2, CO_2, P_2O_5, and SO_3 are the acid anhydrides of sulfurous, carbonic, phosphoric, and sulfuric acids, respectively. Acetic anhydride $(CH_3CO)_2\,O$ reacts with water to form acetic acid.

Acid error: Compare with alkaline error. A systematic error that occurs when glass pH electrodes are used in strongly acidic solutions. Glass electrodes give pH readings that are consistently too high in these solutions.

Acid halide: acid chloride; acyl halide; acyl chloride. Compounds containing a carbonyl group bound to a halogen atom.

Acid-base indicator: A weak acid that has acid and base forms with sharply different colors. Changes in pH around the acid's pKa are "indicated" by color changes.

Acid-base titration: It is a method in pharmaceutical analysis that allows quantitative analysis of the concentration of an unknown acid or base solution.

Acid dissociation constant: (K_a) acid ionization constant. Compare with base hydrolysis constant. The equilibrium constant for the dissociation of an acid into a hydrogen ion and an anion. For example, the acid dissociation constant for acetic acid is the equilibrium constant for $HC_2H_3O_2$ (aq) $\rightleftharpoons$ $H^+(aq) + C_2H_3O_2^-$ (aq), which is $K_a = [H^+][C_2H_3O_2^-]\,/\,[HC_2H_3O_2]$.

Adsorption: adsorb; adsorbed. Compare with absorption and sorption. Adsorption is collection of a substance on the surface of a solid or a liquid. For example, gases that make water taste bad are strongly adsorbed on charcoal granules in water filters.

Adsorption indicator: A substance that indicates an excess of a reactant in a precipitation reaction. For example, dichlorofluorescein is added to NaCl solution being titrated with silver nitrate. Before the endpoint, excess chloride ions make the surface of the AgCl precipitate negative, and dichlorofluorescein anions remain in solution. After the endpoint, the excess silver ions make the surface of the AgCl precipitate positive, and the dichlorofluorescein anions are adsorbed onto their surface. Adsorption changes the color of the indicator from yellow-green to pink.

Alkalimetry titration: It is estimation of acid/acidic drugs by titration with standard alkali.

Alkaline: Having a pH greater than 7.

Amphoteric: Ampholyte. A substance that can act either an acid or a base in a reaction. For example, aluminum hydroxide can neutralize mineral acids ($Al\ (OH)_3 + 3\ HCl = AlCl_3 + 3\ H_2O$) or strong bases ($Al\ (OH)_3 + 3\ NaOH = Na_3AlO_3 + 3\ H_2O$).

Amphiprotic solvent: Compare with aprotic solvent. Solvents that exhibit both acidic and basic properties; amphiprotic solvents undergo autoprotolysis. Examples are water, ammonia, and ethanol.

Analysis: Chemical analysis. Determination of the composition of a sample.

Analyte: An analyte is the sample constituent whose concentration is sought in a chemical analysis.

Aprotic solvent: Compare with amphiprotic solvent. A solvent that does not act as an acid or as a base; aprotic solvents don't undergo autoprotolysis. Examples are pentane, pet ether, and toluene.

Aqua regia: A mixture of nitric and hydrochloric acids, usually 1:3 or 1:4 parts HNO_3 to HCl, used to dissolve gold.

Aqueous: (aq) aqueous solution. A substance dissolved in water

Autoprotolysis: Auto ionization. Transfer of a hydrogen ion between molecules of the same substance, e. g. the autoprotolysis of methanol ($2\ CH_3OH = CH_3OH_2^+ + CH_3O^-$). autoprotolysis of water into hydronium ions and hydroxide ions results in equilibrium concentrations that satisfy $K_w = [H_3O^+][OH^-]$, where the autoprotolysis constant K_w is equal to 1.01×10^{-14} at 25°C.

Amino acid: Amino acids are molecules that contain at least one amine group ($-NH_2$) and at least one carboxylic acid group ($-COOH$). When these groups are both attached to the same carbon, the acid is an α-amino acid. α-amino acids are the basic building blocks of proteins.

Back titration: Indirect titration. Determining the concentration of an analyte by reacting it with a known number of moles of excess reagent. The excess reagent is then titrated with a second reagent. The concentration of the analyte in the original solution is then related to the amount of reagent consumed.

Bidentate: A ligand that has two "teeth" or atoms that coordinates directly to the central atom in a complex. For example, 1,10-phenanthroline is a bidentate ligand of iron.

Base: Alkali; alkaline; basic. Compare with acid. **1.** A compound that reacts with an acid to form a salt. **2.** A compound that produces hydroxide ions in aqueous solution (Arrhenius). **3.** A molecule or ion that captures hydrogen ions. (Bronsted-Lowry). **4.** A molecule or ion that donates an electron pair to form a chemical bond. (Lewis).

Base hydrolysis constant: (K_b) base ionization constant; basic hydrolysis constant. Compare with acid dissociation constant. The equilibrium constant for the hydrolysis reaction associated with a base. For example, K_b for ammonia is the equilibrium constant for NH_3 (aq) + H_2O (l) → NH_4^+ (aq) + OH^-(aq), or $K_b = [NH_4^+][OH^-]/[NH_3]$.

Bronsted acid: Compare with base. A material that gives up hydrogen ions in a chemical reaction.

Bronsted base: Compare with acid. A material that accepts hydrogen ions in a chemical reaction.

Buffer: pH buffer; buffer solution. A solution that can maintain its pH value with little change when acids or bases are added to it. Buffer solutions are usually prepared as mixtures of a weak acid with its own salt or mixtures of salts of weak acids. For example, a 50:50 mixture of 1 M acetic acid and 1 M sodium acetate buffers pH around 4.7.

Burette: A cylindrical glass tube closed by a stopcock on one end and open on the other, with volume gradations marked on the barrel of the tube, used to precisely dispense a measured amount of a liquid.

Calibration: Calibration is correcting a measuring instrument by measuring values whose true values are known. Calibration minimizes systematic error.

Carboxylic acid: Carboxyl; carboxyl group. A carboxylic acid is an organic molecule with a $-(C=O)-OH$ group. The group is also written as $-COOH$ and is called a carboxyl group. The hydrogen on the $-COOH$ group ionizes in water; carboxylic acids are weak acids. The simplest carboxylic acids are formic acid ($H-COOH$) and acetic acid (CH_3-COOH).

Cathode: Compare with anode. The electrode at which reduction occurs.

Cation: Compare with anion. A cation is a positively charged ion. Metals typically form cations.

Chelate: A stable complex of a metal with one or more polydentate ligands. For example, calcium complexes with EDTA to form a chelate.

Chelating agent: chelator. A ligand that binds to a metal using more than one atom; a polydentate ligand.

Colloid: A colloid is a heterogeneous mixture composed of tiny particles suspended in another material. The particles are larger than molecules but less than 1 μm in diameter. Particles this small do not settle out and pass right through filter paper. Milk is an example of a colloid. The particles can be solid, tiny droplets of liquid or tiny bubbles of gas; the suspending medium can be a solid, liquid, or gas (although gas-gas colloids aren't possible).

Common ion effect: The common-ion effect is a term used to describe the effect on a solution of two dissolved solutes that contain the same ion.

Complexing agent: Complexant. A ligand that binds to a metal ion to form a complex.

Complexometric titration: Chelometric titration. A titration based on a reaction between a ligand and a metal ion to form a complex.

For example, free Ca^{2+} in milk powder can be determined by titrating a milk powder sample with EDTA solution, which chelates calcium ion. End point in complexometric titrations are often determined using organochromic indicators.

Complex ion: An ion formed by combination of simpler ions or molecules; for example, Co^{2+} combines with six molecules of water to form the complex ion $Co(H_2O)_6^{2+}$.

Component

1. A substance whose concentration must be specified to describe the state of a mixture in which reactions are occurring.
2. A substance present in a mixture in which no reactions occur.

Compound: Compare with element and mixture. A compound is a material formed from elements chemically combined in definite proportions by mass. For example, water is formed from chemically bound hydrogen and oxygen. Any pure water sample contains 2 g of hydrogen for every 16 g of oxygen.

Concentration: Compare with dilution.

1. A measure of the amount of substance present in a unit amount of mixture. The amounts can be expressed as moles, masses, or volumes.
2. The process of increasing the amount of substance in a given amount of mixture.

Conjugate pairs: A pair of substance which can be formed from one another by the gain or lose of proton are called as conjugate pairs, if the pairing is between acid and base, it is known as acid-base conjugate pairs.

Coordination number: The number of bonds formed by the central atom in a metal-ligand complex.

Co-precipitation: Precipitation of any soluble or extraneous substance along with the precipitate is called as co-precipitation.

Diazonium salt: A diazonium salt is a compound with general form $Ar-NN^+X^-$, where Ar represents a substituted benzene ring and X⁻ is a halide ion such as chloride. Diazonium salts are unstable and explosive in dry form. They are used to manufacture many different organic compounds, including azo dyes.

Diazotization: Diazotization is a reaction that converts an $-NH_2$ group connected to a phenyl ring to a diazonium salt. For example, Diazotization reactions are extremely useful in organic synthesis. The nitrous acid provides NO^+ which replaces a hydrogen on the $-NH_3^+$ group to produce $-NH_2NO^+$ and water; a second water is eliminated to produce the $-N_2^+$ group.

Dichloromethane: Dichloromethane (CH_2Cl_2) is an organic solvent often use to extract organic substances from samples. It is toxic but much less than chloroform or carbon tetrachloride, which were previously used for this purpose.

Differential thermal analysis: (DTA) A technique that is often used to analyze materials that react or decompose at higher temperatures. The difference in temperature between the sample and an inert reference material is monitored as both are heated in a furnace. Phase transitions and chemical reactions taking place in the sample on heating cause the temperature difference to become larger, at temperatures that are characteristic of the sample.

EDTA: Ethylenediamine tetraacetic acid; A polydentate ligand that tightly complexes certain metal ions. EDTA is used as a blood preservative by complexing free calcium ion (which promotes blood clotting). EDTA's ability to bind to lead ions makes it useful as an antidote for lead poisoning.

Electrochemical cell electric cell: A device that uses a redox reaction to produce electricity, or a device that uses electricity to drive a redox reaction in the desired direction.

Electrolytic cell: A device that uses electricity from an external source to drive a redox reaction.

Electrolysis: The process of driving a redox reaction in the reverse direction by passage of an electric current through the reaction mixture.

Endpoint: Compare with equivalence point. The experimental estimate of the equivalence point in a titration. The equivalence point is the point in a titration when enough titrant has been added to react completely with the analyte.

Equivalent: Compare with normality.
1. The amount of substance that gains or loses one mole of electrons in a redox reaction.
2. The amount of substances that releases or accepts one mole of hydrogen ions in a neutralization reaction.
3. The amount of electrolyte that carries one mole of positive or negative charge, for example, 1 mole of Ba^{2+}(aq) is 2 equivalents of Ba^{2+}(aq).

Equivalent weight (EW): The equivalent weight of a substance is defined as the parts by weight of that substance which is chemically equivalent to 1.008 parts by weight of hydrogen or 8 parts by weight of oxygen or 35.45 parts by weight of chlorine.

Experiment: An experiment is direct observation under controlled conditions. Most experiments involve carefully changing one variable and observing the effect on another variable (for example, changing temperature of a water sample and recording the change volume that results).

Fajan's method: This method employs adsorption indicators for the detection of end point in precipitation titrations.

Ferroin: A blood-red complex of Fe^{2+} ion with 1,10-phenanthroline, used as a redox indicator. Ferroin changes from red to pale blue when oxidized.

Formula weight: Formula mass. Compare with molecular weight and empirical formula. The formula weight is the sum of the atomic weights of the atoms in an empirical formula. Formula weights are usually written in atomic mass units (u).

Gay lussac method: It is the method for the determination of end point in argentometric titrations without the use of indicators.

Gram equivalent: It is the number of grams of the substance chemically equivalent to 1 gram-atom (or gram-ion) of hydrogen in a given reaction.

Gravimetry: It involves the separation of the constituents to be estimated in the form of an insoluble precipitate. The insoluble precipitate is washed to free it from all impurities, dried and weighed either as such or ignited to leave a residue of some other compound which is then weighed.

Gross error: Compare with systematic error, random error and mistake. Gross errors are undetected mistakes that cause a measurement to be very much farther from the mean measurement than other measurements.

Hydrolysis: Reaction of a compound with water to form new substance. A catch-all term for any reaction in which the water molecule is split.

Hydronium ion: (H_3O^+) hydronium. The H_3O^+ ion, formed by capture of a hydrogen ion by a water molecule. A strong covalent bond is formed between the hydrogen ion and water oxygen; all hydrogen ions in aqueous solution are bound inside hydronium ions

Hygroscopic: Able to absorb moisture from air. For example, sodium hydroxide pellets are so hygroscopic that they absorb water from the air.

Iodimetry: The titrations with a standards solution of Iodine is refered to as Iodimetry.

Iodometry: It deals with the titrations of Iodine liberated in conical reactions.

Ionic dissociation: ionize; ionization. When ionic substances dissolve, their ions are surrounded by solvent molecules and separated from each other. This phenomena is also called ionization.

Indicator: A substance that undergoes an sharp, easily observable change when conditions in its solutions change.

K_w: Symbol for the autoprotolysis constant for water, equal to 1.01×10^{-14} at 25°C.

Law of mass action: This law states as; "the rate of chemical reactions is directly proportional to the product of 'active masses 'of the reactants".

Ligand
1. In inorganic chemistry, a molecule or ion that binds to a metal cation to form a complex.
2. In biochemistry, a molecule that binds to a receptor, having a biological effect.

Litmus: A mixture of pigments extracted from certain lichens that turns blue in basic solution and red in acidic solution.

Litmus paper: Litmus test. Paper impregnated with litmus, usually cut in narrow strips. Dipping red litmus paper into a basic solution turns it blue; dipping blue litmus paper into an acidic solution turns it red.

Mass percentage: [(w/w)%]. Mass percentages express the concentration of a component in a mixture or an element in a compound. For example, household bleach is 5.25% NaOCl by mass, meaning that every 100 g of bleach contains 5.25 g of NaOCl. Mass percentage can be calculated as 100% times the mass of a component divided by the mass of the mixture containing the component.

Mohr's method: The substance in solution is directly titrated with a titrant or precipitant and end point in the precipitation is determined by the use of internal indicator.

Molality (m): Compare with molarity. Concentration measured as moles of solute per kilogram of solvent. For example, a 1 m NaCl solution contains 1 mole of NaCl per kilogram of water. Molalities are preferred over molarities in experiments that involve temperature changes of solutions, e.g., calorimetry and freezing point depression experiments.

Molar
1. Of or pertaining to moles.
2. An synonym for molarity; for example, a "six molar solution of hydrochloric acid" contains 6 moles of HCl per liter of solution.

Molar volume: The volume occupied by one mole of a material. For example, the molar volume of an ideal gas at STP is 22.4 L/mol.

Molarity (M): Molar concentration. Concentration of a solution measured as the number of moles of solute per liter of solution. For example, a 6 M HCl solution contains 6 moles of HCl per liter of solution.

Mole (mol): SI unit for amount of substance, defined as the number of atoms in exactly 12 g of carbon-12. One mole of a molecular compound contains Avogadro's number molecules and has a mass equal to the substance's molecular weight, in grams.

Mole fraction: Concentration of a substance in a mixture measured as moles of the substance per mole of mixture. For example, the mole fraction of oxygen in air is about 0.21, which means that 1 mol of air contains about 0.21 moles of O_2.

Molecular equation: Compare with ionic equation. A molecular equation is a balanced chemical equation in which ionic compounds are written as neutral formulas rather than as ions. For example, $AgNO_3(aq) + NaCl(aq) = AgCl(s) + NaNO_3(aq)$ is a molecular equation; $Ag^+(aq) + NO_3^-(aq) + Na^+(aq) + Cl^-(aq) = AgCl(s) + Na^+(aq) + NO_3^-(aq)$ is not.

Molecular formula: formula; chemical formula. Compare with empirical formula. A notation that indicates the type and number of atoms in a molecule. The molecular formula of glucose is $C_6H_{12}O_6$, which indicates that a molecule of glucose contains 6 atoms of carbon, 12 atoms of hydrogen, and 6 atoms of oxygen.

Molecular weight: molecular mass. Compare with formula weight and molecular formula. The average mass of a molecule, calculated by summing the atomic weights of atoms in the molecular formula. Note that the words mass and weight are often used interchangeably in chemistry.

Monodentate: A ligand that has only one atom that coordinates directly to the central atom in a complex. For example, ammonia and chloride ion are monodentate ligands of copper in the complexes $[Cu(NH_3)_6]^{2+}$ and $[CuCl_6]^{2+}$.

Nernst equation: The equation gives the relationship between oxidation potential (E) of any given redox system & concentration of oxidized and reduced forms.

Neutral
1. Having no net electrical charge. Atoms are electrically neutral; ions are not.
2. A solution containing equal concentrations of H^+ and OH^-.

Neutralization reaction: Neutralization; acid-base reaction. A chemical change in which one compound acquires H^+ from another. The compound that receives the hydrogen ion is the base; the compound that surrenders it is an acid.

Nitric acid: (HNO_3) aqua fortis. A corrosive liquid with a sharp odor that acts as a strong acid when dissolved in water. Nitric acid is used to synthesize ammonium nitrate for fertilizers, and is also used in the manufacture of explosives, dyes, and pharmaceuticals. Salts of nitric acid are called nitrates.

Non-aqueous titration: Nonaqueous titration is the titration of substances dissolved in nonaqueous solvents.

Normality: Normality (symbol N) is defined as the number of gram equivalents of the solute per litre of solution.

Organic: organic compound. Compare with inorganic compound. Compounds that contain carbon chemically bound to hydrogen. They often contain other elements (particularly O, N, halogens, or S). Organic compounds were once thought to be produced only by living things. We now know that any organic compound can be synthesized in the laboratory (although this can be extremely difficult in practice!)

Oxidation: Oxidize; oxidizing; oxidized. Compare with reduction. Oxidation is the loss of one or more electrons by an atom, molecule, or ion. Oxidation is accompanied by an increase in oxidation number on the atoms, molecules, or ions that lose electrons.

Oxidation half reaction: Compare with reduction half reaction. That part of a redox reaction that involves loss of electrons. In the oxidation half reaction, the oxidation number of one or more atoms within the reactants is increased.

Oxidation number: Oxidation state; positive valence. A convention for representing a charge of an atom embedded within a compound, if the compound were purely ionic. For example, H_2O is a covalent compound; if it was ionic, the hydrogen would be H^+ (oxidation number +1) and the oxygen would be O^{2-} (oxidation number –2). Oxidation number rises for at least one atom in a compound that is oxidized; oxidation number becomes smaller if the compound is reduced.

Oxidizing agent: An agent that gains electrons and is reduced.

Permanganate: (MnO_4^-) permanganate ion. Permanganate ion (MnO_4^-) is a powerful oxidizing agent used in chemical analysis and water treatment. The ion has an intense purple color.

Pharmaceuticals analysis: Pharmaceutical analysis refers to the chemical analysis of drug molecules or medicinal agents and their metabolites.

pH: pH is a measure of effective concentration of hydrogen ions in a solution. It is approximately related to the molarity of H^+ by $pH = -\log [H^+]$.

pH scale: All degrees of acidity and alkalimetry between that of solution moler or normal with respect to H^+ and OH^- ions can be expressed by a series of positive numbers between 0 and 14 in pH scale.

Phenolphthalein: An organic compound used as an acid-base indicator. The compound is colorless in acidic solution and pink in basic solution (with the transition occurring around pH 8.3). Phenolphthalein was used for many years as a laxative in very low concentrations but in high concentrations it is toxic.

pOH: There is also pOH, in a sense the opposite of pH, which measures the concentration of OH^- ions, or the basicity.

Polyprotic systems: Polyprotic systems are compounds that can donate or accept more than one proton.

Potential difference: Electrical potential difference. Work that must be done to move an electric charge between specified points. Electric potential differences are measured in volts.

Precision: Precision is defined at the concordance of a series of measurement of the same quantity.

Precipitate: (↓) ppt. An insoluble substance that has been formed from substances dissolved in a solution. For example, mixing silver nitrate and sodium chloride solutions produces a precipitate, insoluble silver chloride along with soluble sodium nitrate.

Precipitation: Precipitation is the conversion of a dissolved substance into insoluble form by chemical or physical means.

Primary standard: A primary standard is a compound of sufficient purity from which a standard solution can be prepared by direct weighing of a quantity of it.

Proton donor acid: Compare with base. Because a free H^+ ion is technically a bare proton, acids are sometimes referred to as "proton donors" because they release hydrogen ions in solution. The term "proton donor" is misleading, since in aqueous solution, the hydrogen ion is never a bare proton- it's covalently bound to a water molecule as an H_3O^+ ion. Further, acids don't "donate" protons; they yield them to bases with a stronger affinity for them.

Pure substance: A sample of matter that cannot be separated into simpler components without chemical change. Physical changes can alter the state of matter but not the chemical identity of a pure substance. Pure substances have fixed characteristic elemental compositions and properties.

Qualitative analysis: Chemical analysis dealing with the study of nature or quality of the compound or mixture is called qualitative analysis. A chemical analysis that detects the presence of a substance in a sample.

Quantitative analysis: Chemical analysis dealing with the study of determination of how much of each component or of specified compound is present in a given sample. A chemical analysis that determines the concentration of a substance in a sample.

Random error: Indeterminate error. Compare with systematic error, gross error and mistake. Random errors are errors that affect the precision of a set of measurements. Random error scatters measurements above and below the mean, with small random errors being more likely than large ones.

Redox indicator: Oxidation-reduction indicator. An organic molecule that has reduced and oxidized forms with different colors; interconversion of the reduced and oxidized forms of the indicator must be reversible. Ferroin is an example.

Redox reaction: Electrochemical reaction; oxidation-reduction reaction; redox. A reaction that involves transfer of electrons from one substance to another. Redox reactions always involve a change in oxidation number for at least two elements in the reactants.

Redox titration: Oxidation-reduction titration. A titration based on a redox reaction. For example, iron in water can be determined by converting dissolved iron to Fe^{2+} and titrating the solution with potassium permanganate ($KMnO_4$), a powerful oxidizing agent.

Reducing agent: An agent that losses electrons and is oxidized. Compare with oxidizing agent. A reducing agent is a substance that reduce another substance by supplying electrons to it. Reducing agents cause other substances to be reduced in chemical reactions while they themselves are oxidized.

Reduction: Reduce, reduced; reducing. Compare with oxidation. Reduction is gain of one or more electrons by an atom, molecule, or ion. Reduction is accompanied by a decrease in oxidation number.

Reduction half reaction: Reduction half-reaction. Compare with oxidation half reaction. That part of a redox reaction that involves gain of electrons. In the oxidation half reaction, the oxidation number of one or more atoms within the reactants is reduced.

Relative error: Relative uncertainty. Compare with absolute error. The uncertainty in a measurement compared to the size of the measurement. For example, if three replicate weights for an object are 2.00 g, 2.05 g, and 1.95 g, the absolute error can be expressed as ± 0.05 g and the relative error is ± 0.05 g / 2.00 g = 0.025 = 2.5%.

Relative standard deviation: (RSD) Compare with standard deviation. The relative standard deviation is a measure of precision, calculated by dividing the standard deviation for a series of measurements by the average measurement.

Residue

1. The substances left after an evaporation or distillation.

2. A recognizable molecular fragment embedded in a larger molecule; for example, amino acid "residues" within a protein.

Salt bridge: A tube (often filled with ion-laced agar or KBr pellets) that allows two solutions to be in electrical contact without mixing in an electrochemical cell.

Salt hydrolysis: The phenomenon in which a salt reacts with water to produce either acidic or alkaline solution is called salt hydrolysis.

Sampling: The process of withdrawing from the bulk of material, a small portion that is truly representative of the whole material.

Saturated solution: Compare with supersaturated solution. A solution which does not dissolve any more solute. When a saturated solution is placed in contact with additional solute, solute neither dissolves nor is deposited from a saturated solution.

Secondary standard: A secondary standard is a substance which may be used for standardization, and whose content of the active substance has been found by comparison against a primary standard.

Saturated solution: If a solute is added to a solvent with a continuous stirring, firstly solute dissolves and a stage will come when the added solute will not dissolve any more but settles down at the bottom of the container. As this stage solution is called saturated solution.

Significant figures: A significant figure is a digit having some practical meaning i.e. it is a figure or digit which denotes the amount of quantity in the place in which it stands or the digit of a number which are needed to express the precision of the measurements from which the number was derived are known as significant figures.

A convention for recording measurements. Measurements are rounded so that they contain only the digits up to and including the first uncertain digit, when the number is written in scientific notation.

Solubility: Solubilities; equilibrium solubility; solubleness. The solubility of a substance is its concentration in a saturated solution. Substances with solubilities much less than 1 g/100 ml of solvent are usually considered insoluble. The solubility is sometimes called "equilibrium solubility" because the rates at which solute dissolves and is deposited out of solution are equal at this concentration.

Solubility product: (K_{sp}) ion product; solubility product constant; Ksp.
The equilibrium constant for a reaction in which a solid ionic compound dissolves to give its constituent ions in solution. Solubility product of salt is defined as the maximum product of the concentration of its constituent ions in its solution.

Solubilizing group: A group or substructure on a molecule that increases the molecule's solubility. Solubilizing groups usually make the molecule they are attached to ionic or polar. For example, hydrocarbon chains can be made water-soluble by attaching a carboxylic acid group to the molecule.

Soluble: Compare with insoluble. Capable of being dissolved in a solvent (usually water).

Soluble salt: An ionic compound that dissolves in a solvent (usually water).

Strong acid: Compare with weak acid. A strong acid is an acid that completely dissociates into hydrogen ions and anions in solution. Strong acids are strong electrolytes. There are only six common strong acids: HCl (hydrochloric acid), HBr (hydrobromic acid), HI (hydroiodic acid), H_2SO_4 (sulfuric acid), $HClO_4$ (perchloric acid), and HNO_3 (nitric acid).

Strong base: A strong base is a base that completely dissociates into ions in solution. Strong bases are strong electrolytes. The most common strong bases are alkali metal and alkaline earth metal hydroxides.

Sulfuric acid. (H_2SO_4) oil of vitriol; Sulphuric acid. An oily, corrosive liquid that acts as a strong acid when dissolved in water. Sulfuric acid has so many industrial uses that sulfuric acid production was once used as an index of industrial productivity. Salts of sulfuric acids are called sulfates.

Titrant. The substance that quantitatively reacts with the analyte or titrate in a titration. The titrant is usually a standard solution added carefully to the analyte until the reaction is complete. The amount of analyte is calculated from the volume of titrant required for complete reaction.

Titration curve. A plot that summarizes data collected in a titration. A linear titration curve plots moles of analyte (or, some quantity proportional to moles of analyte) on the Y axis, and the volume of titrant added on the X axis. Nonlinear plots use the log of the concentration of the analyte instead. Nonlinear titration curves are often used for neutralization titrations (pH vs. ml NaOH solution). Logs are used to exaggerate the rate of change of concentration on the plot, so that the endpoint can be determined from the point of maximal slope.

Titration. A procedure for determining the amount of some unknown substance (the analyte) by quantitative reaction with a measured volume of a solution of precisely known concentration (the titrant).

Titrimetry. A quantitative method of analysis dealing with the volumes of solution and their measurements is termed as titrimetric analysis.

Universal indicator. It is a pH indicator that has different colors to indicate the range of the pH of the solution it is in or these are blends of different indicators that exhibit several smooth color changes over a wide range of pH values.

Volhard's method: The excess of $AgNO_3$ is added to the solution of halide acidified with nitric acid. The unreacted $AgNO_3$ is treated against standard NH_4CNS solution using ferric salt (Ferric NH_4^+ SO_4^{2-}) as an indicator.

Volume: (V) **1.** The amount of space an object takes up. **2.** The amount of space a container can hold. The SI unit of volume is the cubic meter (m^3); the liter is a popular unit of volume in chemistry.

Volume percentage: ((v/v)%) Volume percentages express the concentration of a component in a mixture or an element in a compound. For example, 95% ethanol by volume contains 95 ml of ethanol in 100 ml of solution.

Volumetry: It is concerned with measuring the volume of gas evolved and absorbed in a chemical method.

Water: (H_2O) dihydrogen monoxide. A colorless, tasteless liquid with some very peculiar properties that stem from the bent H-O-H structure of its molecules.

Weak acid: Compare with strong acid. An acid that only partially dissociates into hydrogen ions and anions in solution. Weak acids are weak electrolytes.

Weak base: Compare with strong base. A base that only partially dissociates into ions in solution. Weak bases are weak electrolytes. Ammonia is an example of a weak base.

Weak electrolyte: Compare with strong electrolyte. A weak electrolyte is a solute that incompletely dissociates into ions in solution. For example, acetic acid partially dissociates into acetate ions and hydrogen ions, so that an acetic acid solution contains both molecules and ions.

Weak ligand: Weak field ligand. Compare with strong field ligand. A ligand that causes a small crystal field splitting which results in a high-spin complex.

Weight: (W) Compare with mass. Weight is the force exerted by an object in a gravitational field. The weight of an object (W) arises from its mass (m): W = mg, where g is the acceleration due to gravity (about 9.8 m/s^2).

Zinc: (Zn). Element 30, atomic weight 65.37, a reactive gray metal that dissolves in acids, used to galvanize metals and in many alloys (e. g. brass and bronze).

Bibliography*

1. Alexeyev .V. *Quantitative Analysis.* 2nd edition, CBS Delhi, 1979.

2. Ali.M, Siddiqui. Anees. A. *Practical Pharmaceutical Chemistry-1,* 1st edition, CBS Delhi, 2006.

3. Bauer. H.H., Christian.G.D, Reilly.J.E. *Instrumental analysis,* Allyn and Bacon, Boston, 1978.

4. Beckett. A.H., Stenlake. J.B. *Practical pharmaceutical chemistry,* 4th edition, CBS Delhi, 2005.

5. Devala. G. *A text book of pharmaceutical analysis-1,* 3rd edition, Birla, Delhi, 2007.

6. Higuchi T., Brochmann-Hanssen. E. *Pharmaceutical Analysis,* Interscience, New York, 1961.

7. Kamboj. P.C. *Pharmaceutical analysis,* 2nd edition, Vallabh, Delhi, 2007.

8. Kenneth. A. Connors. *A text book of pharmaceutical analysis,* 2nd edition, Wiley Interscience, 2004.

9. Kolthoff. I.M., Sandell.E.B, Meehan. E.J., Bruckenstein. *Quantitative chemical analysis,* Macmillan Company, New York, 1969.

10. Mendham. J., Denney. R.C., Barnes. J.D. *Vogel's text book of quantitative chemical analysis,* 6th edition, Dorling Kindersley, India, 2006.

11. Parimoo. P. *Pharmaceutical analysis,* 2nd edition, CBS Delhi, 2005.

(241)

12. Pieper. J.A., Rutledge. D.R. *Current Concepts - Laboratory techniques for pharmacists*, Upjohn, Kalamazoo, 1989.

13. Siddiqui .Anees.A. *Pharmaceutical Analysis*, 1st edition, CBS Delhi, 2006.

14. Singhal.N. Singhal .S. *Fundamentals of Pharmaceutical analysis*, 3rd edition, Pragati Prakashan, Meerut, 2007.

15. Smith. R.V., Stewart. J.T., *Textbook of Biopharmaceutic Analysis*, Lea and Febiger, Philadelphia, 1981.

*Note: The text of this book has been prepared by taking reference from the following editions of various authors.

Index